Organ Printing (Second Edition)

Online at: https://doi.org/10.1088/978-0-7503-5122-5

IPEM–IOP Series in Physics and Engineering in Medicine and Biology

About the Series

The series in Physics and Engineering in Medicine and Biology will allow the Institute of Physics and Engineering in Medicine (IPEM) to enhance its mission to 'advance physics and engineering applied to medicine and biology for the public good'.

It is focused on key areas including, but not limited to:

- clinical engineering
- diagnostic radiology
- informatics and computing
- magnetic resonance imaging
- nuclear medicine
- physiological measurement
- radiation protection
- radiotherapy
- rehabilitation engineering
- ultrasound and non-ionising radiation.

A number of IPEM–IOP titles are being published as part of the EUTEMPE Network Series for Medical Physics Experts.

A full list of titles published in this series can be found here: https://iopscience.iop.org/bookListInfo/physics-engineering-medicine-biology-series.

Organ Printing (Second Edition)

Jinah Jang
Department of Mechanical Engineering, Pohang University of Science and Technology (POSTECH), Pohang, Republic of Korea

Suhun Chae
EDmicBio Inc., Seoul, Republic of Korea

Jungbin Yoon
Department of Mechanical Engineering, Pohang University of Science and Technology (POSTECH), Pohang, Republic of Korea

Hyeonji Kim
Department of Mechanical Engineering, Pohang University of Science and Technology (POSTECH), Pohang, Republic of Korea

Wonbin Park
Department of Mechanical Engineering, Pohang University of Science and Technology (POSTECH), Pohang, Republic of Korea

IOP Publishing, Bristol, UK

ISBN 978-0-7503-5122-5 (ebook)
ISBN 978-0-7503-5120-1 (print)
ISBN 978-0-7503-5123-2 (myPrint)
ISBN 978-0-7503-5121-8 (mobi)

DOI 10.1088/978-0-7503-5122-5

Version: 20231101

IOP ebooks

British Library Cataloguing-in-Publication Data: A catalogue record for this book is available from the British Library.

Published by IOP Publishing, wholly owned by The Institute of Physics, London

IOP Publishing, No.2 The Distillery, Glassfields, Avon Street, Bristol, BS2 0GR, UK

US Office: IOP Publishing, Inc., 190 North Independence Mall West, Suite 601, Philadelphia, PA 19106, USA

Dedicated to the biomedical engineering and biotechnology community.

Contents

Preface

Since the publication of our first edition, the interest in the field of organ printing has significantly expanded. Organ printing, which uses three-dimensional (3D) printing approaches, offers intriguing opportunities for creating complex 3D biological structures. As an unrivaled multidisciplinary technology, 3D bioprinting can facilitate innovative advances in tissue engineering and regenerative medicine. In particular, 3D bioprinting has emerged as a vital tool for developing tissue/organ equivalents with structural and functional resemblance of their native counterparts, which can overcome the limitations of conventional biofabrication methods. Owing to its ability to precisely place living cells with biomaterials and growth factors in a defined and organized manner, 3D bioprinting exhibits significant potential for fulfilling the demands of organ shortages, engineering tissues and organs for regenerative therapy, and building reliable *in vitro* tissue models for drug screening.

Organ printing has evolved with significant advances in 3D printing techniques. Several 3D bioprinting systems have been developed, which can be broadly categorized as inkjet-, extrusion-, or light-based techniques according to their working principles. Recently, more advanced techniques have been proposed to improve the scalability and resolution. Several bioprinting modalities are readily available, each with its distinct characteristics and specific requirements for constructing various tissue types. The use of multiscale and multimaterial fabrication processes in 3D bioprinting is useful for achieving a solid tissue/organ with high levels of structural complexity and physiological function. With the development of bioprinting modalities, diverse cell sources and biomaterials have also evolved. Biomimetic tissue engineering requires significant consideration of the biological requirements and environmental factors, such as the type and arrangement of printed cells, to provide appropriate bioactive cues tailored to the diverse properties of the target tissue. In this context, selection and design of cell sources and printable ink materials are the crucial steps in 3D bioprinting. Significant research has been conducted on 3D bioprinting approaches over the past decade. Organ printing is primarily used in the development of 3D biomimetic tissue constructs as regenerative implants for various tissue engineering applications. In recent years, considerable attention has been focused on the development of *in vitro* models of various tissues to investigate human pathophysiology and predict human responses to therapeutic drugs. Therefore, 3D bioprinting is expected to become the next-generation technology for the production of complex human tissues/organs for clinical translation.

In summary, organ printing has made a significant leap forward in the fields of tissue engineering and regenerative medicine. The primary goal of the second edition is to expand upon the original content, continuing to provide a comprehensive overview of the state-of-the-art 3D bioprinting technologies. This book provides technical perspectives and academic interests on organ printing to non-specialist readers.

Jinah Jang, POSTECH, Republic of Korea
July 2023

Acknowledgements

This work was supported by funded by the National Research Foundation of South Korea (NRF) grant funded by the Ministry of Science and ICT (No. 2021R1A2C2004981 and No.2022R1A2C3004300). This work was supported by Korean Fund for Regenerative Medicine funded by Ministry of Science and ICT, and Ministry of Health and Welfare (No. 21A0104L1). This work was supported by the Korea Institute for Advancement of Technology (KIAT) and the Ministry of Trade, Industry & Energy(MOTIE) of the Republic of Korea (No. P0021109).

Author biographies

Jinah Jang

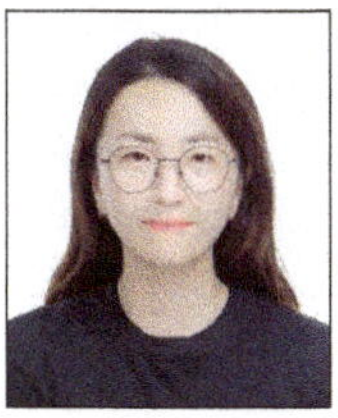

Professor Jinah Jang received her PhD at Pohang University of Science and Technology (POSTECH) in Korea, and trained as postdoctoral fellow in POSTECH and Institute for Stem Cell and Regenerative Medicine at University of Washington. She has joined the POSTECH in 2017 and now an Associate Professor in the Convergence IT Engineering, Mechanical Engineering, and School of Interdisciplinary Bioscience and Bioengineering. She has published more than 110 peer-reviewed articles in prestigious journals in the area of bioprinting and tissue engineering. Her h-index and citations are 42 and more than 8,270, respectively (by Google Scholar). She currently serves as the Associate Editor of Bio-Design and Manufacturing and as an Executive board of directors (Secretary General) for International Society for Biofabrication. She also has received numerous awards including the SME 2022 Sandra L. Bouckley Outstanding Young Engineer Award (2022), and Korea Tissue Engineering and Regenerative Medicine Society (2021). Her research interest lies in engineering the functional human tissues using high-performance stem cells and printable biomaterials-based 3D bioprinting technology.

Suhun Chae

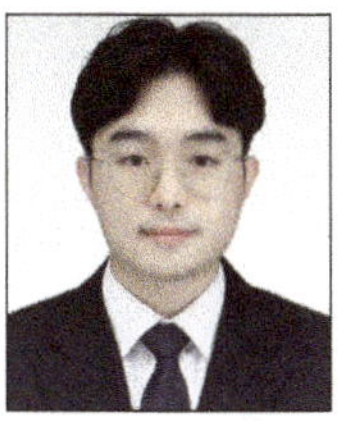

Dr Suhun Chae is a research team director at EDmicBio Inc. He received his bachelor's degree from the Department of Mechanical Engineering, Sogang University in 2015, and completed his PhD in Mechanical Engineering at POSTECH in 2021. His current research interests include 3D bioprinting of organ-on-a-chip platforms and their commercialization for research use.

Jungbin Yoon

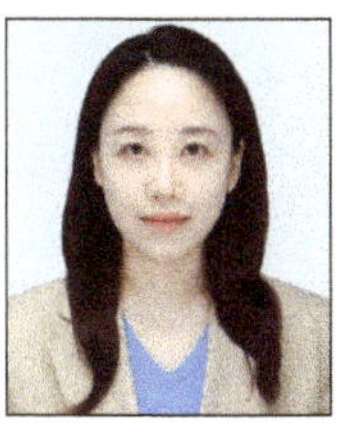

Dr Jungbin Yoon is a research professor at the Department of Mechanical Engineering at POSTECH. She received her bachelor's degree from the Faculty of Arts and Science at the University of Toronto in 2011. She completed her PhD at the School of Biological Sciences at Seoul National University in 2019. Her current research interests include developing an integrative multi-organ-on-a-chip by utilizing multi-biofabrication techniques, including 3D bioprinting technology and tissue-specific bioinks.

Hyeonji Kim

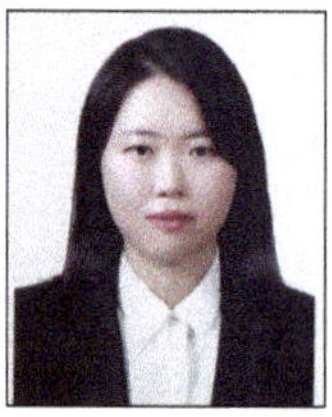

Dr Hyeonji Kim is a research professor in the Department of Mechanical Engineering at POSTECH. She earned her bachelor's degree and completed her PhD in the Department of Mechanical Engineering at POSTECH in 2013 and 2020, respectively. Her present research focus encompasses 3D bioprinting of human-scale tissue and organ equivalents, as well as the advancement of regenerative medicine utilizing tissue-specific bioinks.

Wonbin Park

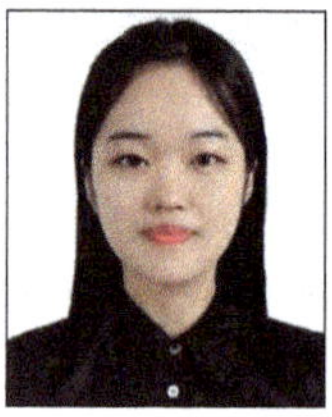

Wonbin Park is a PhD student in the Department of Mechanical Engineering at POSTECH under the guidance of Professor Dong-Woo Cho. She received her bachelor's degree from the Department of Molecular Biology at Pusan National University in 2018. Her current research focuses on the development of in vitro blood vessel models, in vitro metastatic cancer models, and tissue-engineered vascular grafts using 3D bioprinting technology and tissue-derived extracellular matrix bioinks.

Contributors

Jinah Jang
Department of Mechanical Engineering, POSTECH, Pohang, Republic of Korea

Suhun Chae
EDmicBio Inc., Seoul, Republic of Korea

Jungbin Yoon
Department of Mechanical Engineering, POSTECH, Pohang, Republic of Korea

Hyeonji Kim
Department of Mechanical Engineering, POSTECH, Pohang, Republic of Korea

Wonbin Park
Department of Mechanical Engineering, POSTECH, Pohang, Republic of Korea

IOP Publishing

Organ Printing (Second Edition)

Jinah Jang, Suhun Chae, Jungbin Yoon, Hyeonji Kim and Wonbin Park

Chapter 1

Introduction

The continuing demand for organ transplantation and repair, together with a lack of available donors, necessitates the development of innovative strategies to overcome these medical challenges [1]. Organ printing has raised hopes for the development of artificial bioconstructs that can address organ shortage. Organ printing is performed using three-dimensional (3D) bioprinting technologies, which have opened a promising avenue for fabricating tissue/organ analogs [2]. 3D bioprinting involves the precise deposition of living cells using biological materials and growth factors in compliance with a predefined spatial pattern. Over the last few decades, significant advances in 3D bioprinting have been made in the engineering of 3D complex tissue structures for applications in tissue engineering and regenerative medicine [3–5]. With the convergence of different disciplines, including engineering, biology, material science, and medicine, 3D bioprinting has become a powerful tool for the production of a specific 3D functional unit of human tissues and organs, allowing researchers to unveil the fundamental biological processes in tissue development and physiology or provide a new therapeutic solution.

As a core biofabrication technology, different types of bioprinting modalities are currently available for biomanufacturing of functional tissues and organs. According to their working principle, 3D bioprinting techniques can be classified into three main categories: (1) inkjet-, (2) extrusion-, and (3) light-based techniques. With the growing need for improved printing scale and resolution, significant efforts have been expended in the development of several novel bioprinting strategies such as sacrificial, embedding, coaxial, microfluidic-based, and volumetric strategies. Each technique has inherent advantages and limitations. The details of the various 3D bioprinting methods are discussed and compared in chapter 2. Through computer-aided design and computer-aided manufacturing approaches, 3D bio-printing technology facilitates the rapid and reproducible creation of scalable and customizable products using biological elements. For successful bioprinting, the architectural, mechanical, biological, and economic aspects of both biofabrication

doi:10.1088/978-0-7503-5122-5ch1

techniques and tissue constructs should be deliberately considered [6]. Accordingly, employing an appropriate bioprinting modality based on the key properties of the targeted tissues/organs it is of paramount importance. We believe that a basic understanding of 3D bioprinting can provide insights into the fundamental principles, techniques, and key elements pertaining to its translational applications. This innovative biofabrication tool is expanding its spectrum and is expected to revolutionize the biomedical and healthcare industries.

The ultimate goal of bioprinting is to produce a functionally viable construct that fully mimics the structural and physiological characteristics of native tissues [7]. Several parameters must be established and optimized, including cell sourcing, biomaterials, printing design, and strategies, which are essential for generating more complex and functional tissues/organs. Multiple biomaterials have been utilized to print functional and viable organs, support 3D structures, and provide bioactive cues to enhance cellular activity. The types of biomaterials vary with different physical and biological properties depending on the desired properties of each organ. Bioink is an essential element in 3D bioprinting. Bioink can be defined as 'a formulation of cells that is suitable to be processed by an automated biofabrication technology' [8]. Hydrogels are preferentially used to formulate bioinks, as they serve as a cell-friendly microenvironment that can modulate cellular behaviors. In this context, the selection of bioinks with optimal rheological and biological properties for successful bioprinting is crucial for maintaining cell viability and stimulating the growth or differentiation of specific cell and tissue types. Cell sourcing is another key parameter becasue tissue printing requires a large number of cells. Because each human tissue or organ consists of different cell types, incorporating tissue-specific cells is imperative for developing biologically functional constructs. Currently, primary cells, stem cells, and organoids are promising sources for the development of 3D bioprinted tissue/organ models [9]. In particular, 3D bioprinting promises significant control over the spatial positioning of multiple cells, mimicking the dimensional and morphological features of target tissues. When tissue building blocks are constructed, the printed cells actively interact and behave similar to those in the native tissue, resulting in the transformation of native tissue-like constructs. Details of the cell sources and bioprintable materials are described in chapters 3 and 4, respectively.

To date, 3D bioprinting offers a possible solution to circumvent the ongoing demand for organ transplantation and the use of animal models in the drug discovery pipeline [10, 11]. A major application of bioprinted constructs is the development of biological substitutes for regenerating impaired tissues. Numerous bioprinting studies have documented the development of tissue-engineered constructs, highlighting their therapeutic potential in promoting healing and tissue repair. Although fully functional bioprinted organs have not yet been achieved, 3D bioprinting exhibits considerable promise for producing whole organs with complex and multifaceted hierarchical organizations in a 3D microenvironment. Recently, bioprinting has been used to construct *in vitro* biological model systems for tissue and disease modeling, drug development, and personalized therapeutic screening [1]. Moreover, 3D bioprinting with high-precision and automated operation contributes to the engineering of advanced 3D *in vitro* models that reproduce the biological and physiological functions of human tissues/organs, enabling the replacement of existing preclinical methods, such as oversimplified cell culture and inherently discrepant animal models. The use of bioprinted tissue models can advance our understanding of the governing mechanisms of disease development and aid in screening potential therapeutic drug candidates. Thus, the engineering of advanced *in vitro* models is expected to be an efficient tool for improving prediction accuracy and to reducing the time and cost of drug discovery and development.

In summary, organ printing has driven major innovations in the fields of tissue engineering and regenerative medicine with the aim of developing living functional constructs for tissue and organ regeneration. In parallel with tissue engineering applications, the usefulness of 3D bioprinting techniques can be expanded to generate *in vitro* tissue and organ models for studying human pathophysiology and discovering new drugs. This new edition intensively delineates the recent developments in 3D bioprinted constructs using advanced biofabrication techniques and smart bioinks for tissue regeneration and modeling. Finally, current challenges and fascinating opportunities are discussed, providing technical and translational perspectives on organ printing.

References

[1] Mota C, Camarero-Espinosa S, Baker M B, Wieringa P and Moroni L 2020 Bioprinting: from tissue and organ development to *in vitro* models *Chem. Rev.* **120** 10547–607

[2] Harley W S, Li C C, Toombs J, O'Connell C D, Taylor H K, Heath D E and Collins D J 2021 Advances in biofabrication techniques towards functional bioprinted heterogeneous engineered tissues: a comprehensive review *Bioprinting* **23** e00147

[3] Li C and Cui W 2021 3D bioprinting of cell-laden constructs for regenerative medicine *Eng. Regen.* **2** 195–205

[4] Zhang B, Gao L, Ma L, Luo Y, Yang H and Cui Z 2019 3D bioprinting: a novel avenue for manufacturing tissues and organs *Engineering* **5** 777–94

[5] Ashammakhi N, Ahadian S, Xu C, Montazerian H, Ko H, Nasiri R, Barros N and Khademhosseini A 2019 Bioinks and bioprinting technologies to make heterogeneous and biomimetic tissue constructs *Mater. Today Bio.* **1** 100008

[6] Daly A C, Prendergast M E, Hughes A J and Burdick J A 2021 Bioprinting for the biologist *Cell* **184** 18–32

[7] Jo Y, Hwang D G, Kim M, Yong U and Jang J 2023 Bioprinting-assisted tissue assembly to generate organ substitutes at scale *Trends Biotechnol.* **41** 93–105

[8] Groll J *et al* 2019 A definition of bioinks and their distinction from biomaterial inks *Biofabrication* **11** 013001

[9] Chua C K 2014 Cell sources for bioprinting *Bioprinting* (Singapore: World Scientific) pp 165–77

[10] Yi H-G, Kim H, Kwon J, Choi Y-J, Jang J and Cho D-W 2021 Application of 3D bioprinting in the prevention and the therapy for human diseases *Signal Transduct. Target. Ther.* **6** 177

[11] Dey M and Ozbolat I T 2020 3D bioprinting of cells, tissues and organs *Sci. Rep.* **10** 14023

IOP Publishing

Organ Printing (Second Edition)

Jinah Jang, Suhun Chae, Jungbin Yoon, Hyeonji Kim and Wonbin Park

Chapter 2

Three-dimensional (3D) bioprinting techniques

As a core biofabrication technology, 3D bioprinting has been extensively applied in the biomedical field and has emerged as an essential tool for tissue engineering, human tissue/disease modeling, and drug screening. Different bioprinting techniques are currently available for developing functional tissues and organs. This technology generates scalable and customizable products using living cells with suitable biomaterials and biomolecules, which ultimately mimics the physical, architectural, and biological properties of native tissues.

2.1 Practical workflow to implement bioprinting

There are several practical steps in implementing bioprinting, including: (1) pre-printing, (2) printing, and (3) post-printing processes. In the pre-printing process, two main aspects must be considered: the design of the printing model and selection of bioinks. Computer-aided-design (CAD) models are often acquired using medical imaging instruments (e.g., computer tomography and magnetic resonance imaging) or CAD drawing software before designing the models. Once CAD models with optimal design are obtained, they can be converted into stereolithography (STL) files to create G-code for generating an automated printing path. Moreover, certain important parameters must be considered when selecting ink materials in the bioprinting planning phase, including printability, crosslinking strategy, and bio-chemical/biophysical properties [1, 2]. In the printing process, bioprinting systems equipped with nozzles and syringes create the desired 3D constructs through the controllable deposition of bioinks. Numerous printing settings (e.g., temperature, nozzle diameter, printing speed, and flow rate) related to functionality, rigidity, and stability must be optimized to ensure successful fabrication [3]. In the post-printing process, the end construct matures in an incubator under certain physiological conditions. In accordance with specific research purposes, practical considerations involve media formulations, culture conditions, and periods. To ameliorate the maturity of bioprinted constructs, custom bioreactor systems may be employed,

doi:10.1088/978-0-7503-5122-5ch2

providing different physical stimuli such as shear stress, hydrostatic pressure, and electromechanical stimuli [4]. Finally, the resulting constructs can be implanted *in vivo* for regenerative medicine or assessed *in vitro* for disease modeling and drug screening.

Tissue-engineered constructs must exhibit several key requirements, including biocompatibility, biodegradability, architectural and compositional heterogeneity akin to native tissues, and long-term structural stability [5, 6]. Conventionally, various biofabrication methods, including freeze-drying, solvent casting/particulate leaching, gas forming, molding, and textile technologies, have been developed to create porous scaffolds [1, 7, 8]. However, they do not completely meet the ideal requirements for engineering functional tissue analogs. Alternatively, 3D bioprinting can build complex tissue structures through the controllable deposition of biological elements in a layer-by-layer manner. This technology offers the benefits of automation, scalability, reproducibility, customization, and cost-effectiveness [9–11]. These features can enable the creation of multicellular and heterogeneous structures that resemble natural tissues/organs in a rapid and reproducible manner.

2.2 Prevailing 3D bioprinting techniques

3D bioprinting techniques are typically divided into three categories based on their working principles: inkjet-, extrusion-, light-based techniques (figure 2.1). Each technique has advantages and inherent drawbacks. The different properties of these techniques should be discussed with respect to the fabrication method, resolution, printing speed, cell viability, and range of viscosities for the applicable biomaterials.

2.2.1 Inkjet-based 3D bioprinting technique

Inkjet-based printing is a non-contact method that utilizes thermal or piezoelectric forces to expel a tiny volume (1–100 pl) of bioink droplets onto a substrate in a drop-on-demand mode (figure 2.1(A)) [12]. Thermal inkjet bioprinting employs a heating element to increase the temperature (typically 200 °C–300 °C) of the printer head, resulting in vaporization while forming bubbles, which are forcefully ejected as droplets of varying sizes [6]. In contrast, piezoelectric inkjet bioprinting uses a piezoelectric actuator to create droplets [13], and rapid deformation of the

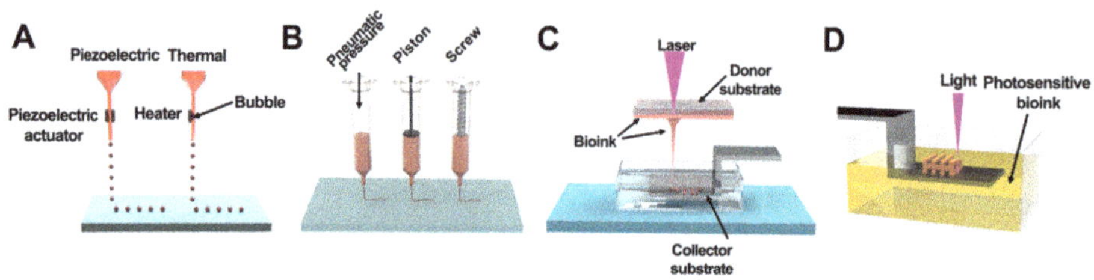

Figure 2.1. Schematic illustration of three-dimensional (3D) bioprinting techniques with different working principles. (A) Inkjet-based printing, (B) extrusion-based printing, (C) and (D) light-based printing, including laser-induced forward transfer (C) and stereolithography (D); Reproduced with permission from [11] CC BY 4.0.

piezoelectric transducer can generate a direct mechanical pulse, resulting in droplet ejection through the nozzle.

The advantage of inkjet-based bioprinting includes low cost, ease-of-use, high printing speed (10 000 droplets/s), resolution (with ~50 μm droplets), and relatively high cell viability (70%–90%), offering a potential tool for tissue engineering applications [14, 15]. However, certain major drawbacks are exhibited when building volumetric 3D structures, primarily because bioinks with low viscosity (~3–12 mPa•s) and low dispensing volume are required [16]. Further limitations include inconsistent droplet sizes, the inability to use high-viscosity materials or cells with high density, and the frequent occurrence of nozzle clogging.

2.2.2 Extrusion-based 3D bioprinting technique

Extrusion-based printing is the most versatile technique that utilizes pneumatic pressure or mechanical forces (piston, or screw drive) for the controllable deposition of ink material in the form of a continuous filament through a nozzle (figure 2.1(B)) [17]. Extrusion-based printing systems are often equipped with one or more cartridges for the selective extrusion of different combinations of cells and biomaterials. In these systems, several printing parameters, such as temperature, flow rate, nozzle size, ink properties, and crosslinking strategies, significantly influence the resulting bioprinted constructs. The key strengths of extrusion bioprinting include the availability of a large pool of applicable bioink types with varying viscosities (30–6 × 10^7 mPa•s) and the ability to print cell spheroids/aggregates or a high density of cells [16, 18]. Among the diverse bioprinting techniques, extrusion-based bioprinting is the most widely used approach for the rapid fabrication of 3D complex tissue structures with multiple cells owing to its simplicity, scalability, multi-material processability, ease of operation, high structural integrity, and affordability [19]. Despite its versatility and widespread use in 3D bioprinting and tissue engineering, this technique poses certain drawbacks. The extrusion process exerts shear stress on cells when being dispensed out of the nozzle, which may impair biofunctionality and cell viability; reportedly, cell viability after extrusion printing reveals a decreasing tendency (40%–86%) and is lower than that of other printing techniques [18, 20]. Moreover, this nozzle-based approach is limited to a relatively low printing resolution of hundredths of micrometers [21].

2.2.3 Light-based 3D bioprinting technique

Light-based bioprinting is a nozzle-free method that harnesses lasers or light source systems to fabricate complex 3D structures. Scaffold-free printing techniques can be divided into two types: (1) laser-assisted methods and (2) stereolithography (SLA). Laser-induced forward transfer (LIFT) is a common type of laser-assisted bioprinting modality that consists of three main modules, including a pulsed laser source, ribbon structure comprising a laser-absorbing layer on the top and a bioink layer placed on the bottom, and collecting substrate (figure 2.1(C)) [22]. In LIFT, pulsed laser beams are initially illuminated and delivered through the absorbing layer of the ribbon where the focal point of the laser induces local evaporation and generates high-pressure bubbles, thereby depositing bioink droplets onto the collecting substrate [23]. The SLA system uses ultraviolet (UV), infrared, or visible light to solidify the photo-sensitive bioinks point-by-point in a predesigned pattern (figure 2.1(D)). SLA can create selective cell patterning of intricate 3D geometries with sub-micrometer resolution through a layer-by-layer method [24].

The primary advantages of this nozzle-free and non-contact approach lie in the elimination of nozzle clogging and the absence of harsh shear stress on the cells during the printing process, resulting in relatively high cell viability (>85%) and high spatial resolution (~1 m) [23, 25]. Moreover, it allows the use of cells with high concentration or highly viscous materials to form 3D objects/tissues. However, the major limitation of this technique is the potential cell damage due to the exposure to intense UV radiation, which impedes its widespread adoption for cell-laden tissue fabrication.

2.3 Advanced 3D bioprinting techniques

Despite significant advancements in 3D bioprinting techniques, formidable challenges remain in the development of complex, heterogeneous tissue constructs with greater accuracy. Recently, several advanced bioprinting strategies have been proposed to overcome the problems pertaining to scalablity and resolution.

Sacrificial bioprinting is performed using extrusion-based bioprinting, where dissolvable 'fugitive' ink materials are deposited in any desired geometry to provide temporary support during the printing process. Following the casting of the cell-laden or secondary hydrogel, the removal of the sacrificial templates (fugitive ink layers) achieves the generation of 3D interconnected hollow microchannels of arbitrary structures with high connectivity that can be perfused or seeded with cells. This indirect method has been widely explored for the development of 3D vascularized tubular networks [26–28]. Sacrificial bioprinting offers advantages such as a high degree of design freedom for channel geometries at various scales. However, in this method, the channel resolution largely depends on the nozzle diameter, limiting its use in capturing complex microscale vascular networks such as capillary vessels.

Freeform reversible embedding of suspended hydrogels (FRESH) bioprinting involves an extrusion-based embedding approach for printing soft hydrogels into a liquid support bath, where the liquid bath serves as a temporary, thermoreversible, and biocompatible support to retain the printed bioinks in place until stabilization [29]. The FRESH technique enhances the geometrical complexity of bioprinted tissue constructs from low-viscosity ink materials, enabling the direct printing of 3D volumetric structures [29, 30]. Moreover, FRESH can significantly improve the printing resolution (ranging from a few millimeters to centimeters) and enable the use of a larger variety of soft bioinks with high shape fidelity to better mimic tissue complexity.

Coaxial bioprinting utilizes a core/shell printing configuration comprising two needles in a coaxial arrangement, enabling the simultaneous flow of two entirely separated fluids. This technique enables the production of complex tubular structures that are layered with different bioinks with respect to the design of different nozzle constituents. Owing to its simplicity, scalability, and versatility, coaxial bioprinting has been extensively used for creating vascular constructs [31–33]. Different materials can be dispensed through the inner and outer nozzles in coaxial mode, resulting in a more convenient method for the printing of multilayered hollow structures [6]. The key advantage of this technique is its ability to control the organization of internal and external hierarchical geometries in a single process.

Microfluidics-based bioprinting implements a microfluidic device that is applied to the dispensing head in an extrusion system to rapidly and accurately switch between different bioinks and patterns [34]. Using a microfluidic system in the printing head, the fluid flow of different bioinks can be manipulated in a significantly defined and controlled manner, resulting in dispensing multiple bioinks from one nozzle [35, 36]. The integration of extrusion 3D bioprinting with a microfluidic system has allowed the utilization of a wide range of bioinks with varying viscosities, as well as fabrication of complex, heterogeneous 3D structures with high shape fidelity and accuracy [35, 37, 38].

Volumetric bioprinting is a light-based printing approach that uses digital light projection (DLP) strategies. Unlike SLA, DLP-based volumetric bioprinting exploits tomographic light projections that simultaneously elicit the single-step polymerization of a complete layer, leading to the generation of a 3D object within tens of seconds [39, 40]. This printing method facilitates the ultrafast fabrication of 3D complex structures with greater structural integrity and mechanical properties. Furthermore, it allows the use of biocompatible hydrogels for the highly accurate printing of anatomical structures. Volumetric bioprinting exhibits certain advantages in terms of printing speed, resolution (~40 μm), and upscaling capability [40–42]. However, this technique is still in its infancy, and further investigations, including but not limited to the range of applicable biomaterials and the introduction of cell types, are required.

2.4 Conclusion

The ultimate aim of 3D bioprinting is to produce 3D biomimetic tissue/organ analogs with superior cell viability and structural accuracy. Three practical steps in the 3D bioprinting process are introduced, and the important considerations in each bioprinting phase are described. Furthermore, the working principles and features of multiple bioprinting techniques are discussed. Notably, an immaculate technique that concurrently possesses all the aforementioned benefits does not exist. Therefore, given the unique characteristics of each bioprinting method, researchers are compelled to establish effective biofabrication strategies by choosing adequate techniques (alone or in combination) for ideal 3D bioprinting of physiologically relevant tissues and organs.

2.5 End-of chapter problem and examples

Q1. Describe the general steps of 3D bioprinting.

A. The 3D bioprinting process consists of three general steps: (1) pre-printing to design tissue/organ models and select ink materials, (2) printing the designed construct, and (3) post-printing process to culture the bioprinted constructs for maturation, which can be implanted *in vivo* or evaluated *in vitro* for disease modeling/drug screening.

Q2. Describe the ultimate goal of 3D bioprinting in tissue engineering and regenerative medicine.

A. The ultimate goal of 3D bioprinting is to develop 3D complex organs that can fully replicate native tissue structure and function.

References

[1] Yu J, Park S A, Kim W D, Ha T, Xin Y-Z, Lee J and Lee D 2020 Current advances in 3d bioprinting technology and its applications for tissue engineering *Polymers* **12** 2958

[2] Mota C, Camarero-Espinosa S, Baker M B, Wieringa P and Moroni L 2020 Bioprinting: from tissue and organ development to *in vitro* models *Chem. Rev.* **120** 10547–607

[3] Daly A C, Prendergast M E, Hughes A J and Burdick J A 2021 Bioprinting for the biologist *Cell* **184** 18–32

[4] Castro N, Ribeiro S, Fernandes M M, Ribeiro C, Cardoso V, Correia V, Minguez R and Lanceros-Mendez S 2020 Physically active bioreactors for tissue engineering applications *Adv. Biosyst.* **4** 2000125

[5] Chae S and Cho D-W 2023 Biomaterial-based 3D bioprinting strategy for orthopedic tissue engineering *Acta Biomater.* **156** 4–20

[6] Gu Z, Fu J, Lin H and He Y 2020 Development of 3D bioprinting: from printing methods to biomedical applications *Asian J. Pharm. Sci.* **15** 529–57

[7] Pedde R D *et al* 2017 Emerging biofabrication strategies for engineering complex tissue constructs *Adv. Mater.* **29** 1606061

[8] Ning Z and Xiongbiao C 2013 Biofabrication of tissue scaffolds ed P Rosario *Advances in Biomaterials Science and Biomedical Applications* (Rijeka: IntechOpen) ch 12

[9] Chae S and Cho D-W 2022 Three-dimensional bioprinting with decellularized extracellular matrix-based bioinks in translational regenerative medicine *MRS Bull.* **47** 70–9

[10] Atala A and Forgacs G 2019 Three-dimensional bioprinting in regenerative medicine: reality, hype, and future *Stem Cells Transl. Med.* **8** 744–5

[11] Yi H-G, Kim H, Kwon J, Choi Y-J, Jang J and Cho D-W 2021 Application of 3D bioprinting in the prevention and the therapy for human diseases *Signal Transduct. Target. Ther.* **6** 177

[12] Saunders R E and Derby B 2014 Inkjet printing biomaterials for tissue engineering: bioprinting *Int. Mater. Rev.* **59** 430–48

[13] Lorber B, Hsiao W-K, Hutchings I M and Martin K R 2014 Adult rat retinal ganglion cells and glia can be printed by piezoelectric inkjet printing *Biofabrication* **6** 015001

[14] Harley W S, Li C C, Toombs J, O'Connell C D, Taylor H K, Heath D E and Collins D J 2021 Advances in biofabrication techniques towards functional bioprinted heterogeneous engineered tissues: a comprehensive review *Bioprinting* **23** e00147

[15] Zhang X and Zhang Y 2015 Tissue engineering applications of three-dimensional bioprinting *Cell Biochem. Biophys.* **72** 777–82

[16] Hölzl K, Lin S, Tytgat L, Van Vlierberghe S, Gu L and Ovsianikov A 2016 Bioink properties before, during and after 3D bioprinting *Biofabrication* **8** 032002

[17] Weng T *et al* 2021 3D bioprinting for skin tissue engineering: current status and perspectives *J. Tissue Eng.* **12** 20417314211028574

[18] Murphy S V and Atala A 2014 3D bioprinting of tissues and organs *Nat. Biotechnol.* **32** 773–85

[19] Ozbolat I T and Hospodiuk M 2016 Current advances and future perspectives in extrusion-based bioprinting *Biomaterials* **76** 321–43

[20] Chang R, Nam J and Sun W 2008 Effects of dispensing pressure and nozzle diameter on cell survival from solid freeform fabrication–based direct cell writing *Tissue Eng. Part* A **14** 41–8

[21] Liu W *et al* 2017 Rapid continuous multimaterial extrusion bioprinting *Adv. Mater.* **29** 1604630

[22] Michael S, Sorg H, Peck C-T, Koch L, Deiwick A, Chichkov B, Vogt P M and Reimers K 2013 Tissue engineered skin substitutes created by laser-assisted bioprinting form skin-like structures in the dorsal skin fold chamber in mice *PLoS One* **8** e57741

[23] Guillotin B *et al* 2010 Laser assisted bioprinting of engineered tissue with high cell density and microscale organization *Biomaterials* **31** 7250–6

[24] Wang Z, Kumar H, Tian Z, Jin X, Holzman J F, Menard F and Kim K 2018 Visible light photoinitiation of cell-adhesive gelatin methacryloyl hydrogels for stereolithography 3D bioprinting *ACS Appl. Mater. Interfaces* **10** 26859–69

[25] Koch L, Gruene M, Unger C and Chichkov B 2013 Laser assisted cell printing *Curr. Pharm. Biotechnol.* **14** 91–7

[26] Kolesky D B, Truby R L, Gladman A S, Busbee T A, Homan K A and Lewis J A 2014 3D bioprinting of vascularized, heterogeneous cell-laden tissue constructs *Adv. Mater.* **26** 3124–30

[27] Lee V K, Kim D Y, Ngo H, Lee Y, Seo L, Yoo S-S, Vincent P A and Dai G 2014 Creating perfused functional vascular channels using 3D bio-printing technology *Biomaterials* **35** 8092–102

[28] Ouyang L, Armstrong J P K, Chen Q, Lin Y and Stevens M M 2020 Void-free 3D bioprinting for *in situ* endothelialization and microfluidic perfusion *Adv. Funct. Mater.* **30** 1908349

[29] Hinton T J, Jallerat Q, Palchesko R N, Park J H, Grodzicki M S, Shue H-J, Ramadan M H, Hudson A R and Feinberg A W 2015 Three-dimensional printing of complex biological structures by freeform reversible embedding of suspended hydrogels *Sci. Adv.* **1** e1500758

[30] Lee A, Hudson A R, Shiwarski D J, Tashman J W, Hinton T J, Yerneni S, Bliley J M, Campbell P G and Feinberg A W 2019 3D bioprinting of collagen to rebuild components of the human heart *Science* **365** 482–7

[31] Gao G *et al* 2017 Tissue engineered bio-blood-vessels constructed using a tissue-specific bioink and 3D coaxial cell printing technique: a novel therapy for ischemic disease *Adv. Funct. Mater.* **27** 1700798

[32] Shao L, Gao Q, Zhao H, Xie C, Fu J, Liu Z, Xiang M and He Y 2018 Fiber-based mini tissue with morphology-controllable GelMA microfibers *Small* **14** 1802187

[33] Zhang Y S *et al* 2016 Bioprinting 3D microfibrous scaffolds for engineering endothelialized myocardium and heart-on-a-chip *Biomaterials* **110** 45–59

[34] du Chatinier D N, Figler K P, Agrawal P, Liu W and Zhang Y S 2021 The potential of microfluidics-enhanced extrusion bioprinting *Biomicrofluidics* **15** 041304

[35] Colosi C, Shin S R, Manoharan V, Massa S, Costantini M, Barbetta A, Dokmeci M R, Dentini M and Khademhosseini A 2016 Microfluidic bioprinting of heterogeneous 3D tissue constructs using low-viscosity bioink *Adv. Mater.* **28** 677–84

[36] Hardin J O, Ober T J, Valentine A D and Lewis J A 2015 Microfluidic printheads for multimaterial 3D printing of viscoelastic inks *Adv. Mater.* **27** 3279–84
[37] Abelseth E, Abelseth L, De la Vega L, Beyer S T, Wadsworth S J and Willerth S M 2019 3D printing of neural tissues derived from human induced pluripotent stem cells using a fibrin-based bioink *ACS Biomater. Sci. Eng.* **5** 234–43
[38] Zhao H *et al* 2018 Airflow-assisted 3D bioprinting of human heterogeneous microspheroidal organoids with microfluidic nozzle *Small* **14** 1802630
[39] Hong H *et al* 2020 Digital light processing 3D printed silk fibroin hydrogel for cartilage tissue engineering *Biomaterials* **232** 119679
[40] Bernal P N, Delrot P, Loterie D, Li Y, Malda J, Moser C and Levato R 2019 Volumetric bioprinting of complex living-tissue constructs within seconds *Adv. Mater.* **31** 1904209
[41] Loterie D, Delrot P and Moser C 2020 High-resolution tomographic volumetric additive manufacturing *Nat. Commun.* **11** 852
[42] Bernal P N *et al* 2022 Volumetric bioprinting of organoids and optically tuned hydrogels to build liver-like metabolic biofactories *Adv. Mater.* **34** 2110054

IOP Publishing

Organ Printing (Second Edition)

Jinah Jang, Suhun Chae, Jungbin Yoon, Hyeonji Kim and Wonbin Park

Chapter 3

Cell sources

Because each human tissue or organ contains different cell types, the integration and encapsulation of tissue-specific cells are essential for creating functional tissue/organ constructs. Thus, primary cells, stem cells, and organoids are significant sources of cells that can be used to build 3D bioprinted tissue/organ models. In particular, 3D bioprinting promises significant control over the spatial positioning of multiple cells in 3D space.

3.1 Primary cells

Most human primary cells (autologous cells) are isolated from tissue biopsies obtained from healthy individuals and patients after *in vitro* expansion. The significant advantages of using patient-derived primary cells for tissue engineering are the absence of immune rejections and further disease transmission. However, isolation and long-term culture of viable primary cells are not easily accessible because of their limited life span and low proliferation potential under *in vitro* conditions [1]. Human liver-derived hepatocyte, which is a type of primary cell, changes cell morphology, structure, polarity, and gene expression and loses its tissue-specific function during two-dimensional (2D) culture [2]. However, after hepatocytes with other supporting fibroblasts and endothelial cells were encapsulated in growth-factor-rich decellularized extracellular matrix (dECM) bioinks for *in vitro* 3D culture, the enhanced viability and functionality of primary cells were sustained for a long time [3].

Moreover, primary proximal tubule epithelial cells and podocytes in kidney-derived dECM bioinks were printed in a 3D tubular architecture to establish *in vitro* 3D kidney models. In such *in vitro* 3D models, the biological functions (maturation, differentiation, proliferation, and cell survival) of primary cells were significantly improved [4, 5].

doi:10.1088/978-0-7503-5122-5ch3

3.2 Stem cells

Recently, stem cells (human induced pluripotent stem cells [iPSCs]) have been used more frequently to fabricate *in vitro* 3D models via 3D bioprinting. Human stem cells maintain self-renewal abilities and properties that allow them to differentiate between the multiple cell types of different lineages. The reprogrammable capability of human stem cells (cellular phenotypic variability) provides unlimited cell sources for tissue engineering. Moreover, human iPSC (patient-specific stem cells) are a promising source for an enhanced understanding of disease mechanisms. When iPSC-derived bioprinted constructs were transplanted into hosts, the stem cells reduced host rejection and boosted tissue repair and regeneration [6].

3.3 Preparation of cells for 3D organ bioprinting

For 3D organ bioprinting, a large number of (highly dense) cells must be encapsulated within a gel-like extracellular matrix (ECM) hydrogel to form a printable bioink. The viability of the encapsulated cells in the ECM bioink (before the printing process) and on 3D biofabricated constructs (after the printing process) must be sustained to establish mature functional tissues *in vitro*. The 0.6%–3% (w/v) ECM bioinks yielded less shear stress and secreted cell proliferation/maturation-favored ECM components [7, 8]. These synergistic interactions between the ECM bioink and cell sources guaranteed over 85% cell viability from printed 3D constructs for seven days [9–11].

3.4 Cell spheroids

For several decades, cell spheroids have been used as *in vitro* 3D modeling systems for biomedical and tumor research. Spheroids are aggregates of one or multiple cell types that have been used to mimic cardiac, hepatic, and tumor cells [12–14]. In 3D bioprinting-based fabrication, spheroids act as building blocks for fabricating volumetric tissues or tumor-relevant microenvironments [15]. Spheroids possess a non-apical cell morphology with stronger cell-to-cell and cell-to-ECM interactions. Initially, spheroids are formed by boosting cell-to-cell interactions while minimizing cell-to-matrix adhesion [16]. Multiple cells aggregate to form loose bonds via integrin-mediated attachment to the ECM, thereby substantiating cadherin upregulation. The accumulation of cadherins on the cell membrane facilitates the formation of compact spheroids [17]. Spheroids also exhibit three zones in the central core: the outer proliferation zone, middle quiescent zone, and innermost necrotic zone [17]. Cells in the proliferation zone receive abundant oxygen and nutrients from the culture medium, resulting in a significantly higher proliferation rate and cell viability. In contrast, cells in the core zone are relatively quiescent or hypoxic because of the lack of oxygen and nutrient supplies [18].

The 'drop-on-demand'-style printing capability for accurately dispensing spheroids makes these techniques appealing for high-throughput spheroid formation (figure 3.1(A)) [19]. By allocating cell droplets into an alginate hydrogel matrix residing within a 96-well plate (enables high-throughput printing by using a bespoke drop-on-demand 3D bioprinter), Utama *et al* successfully generated spheroids using

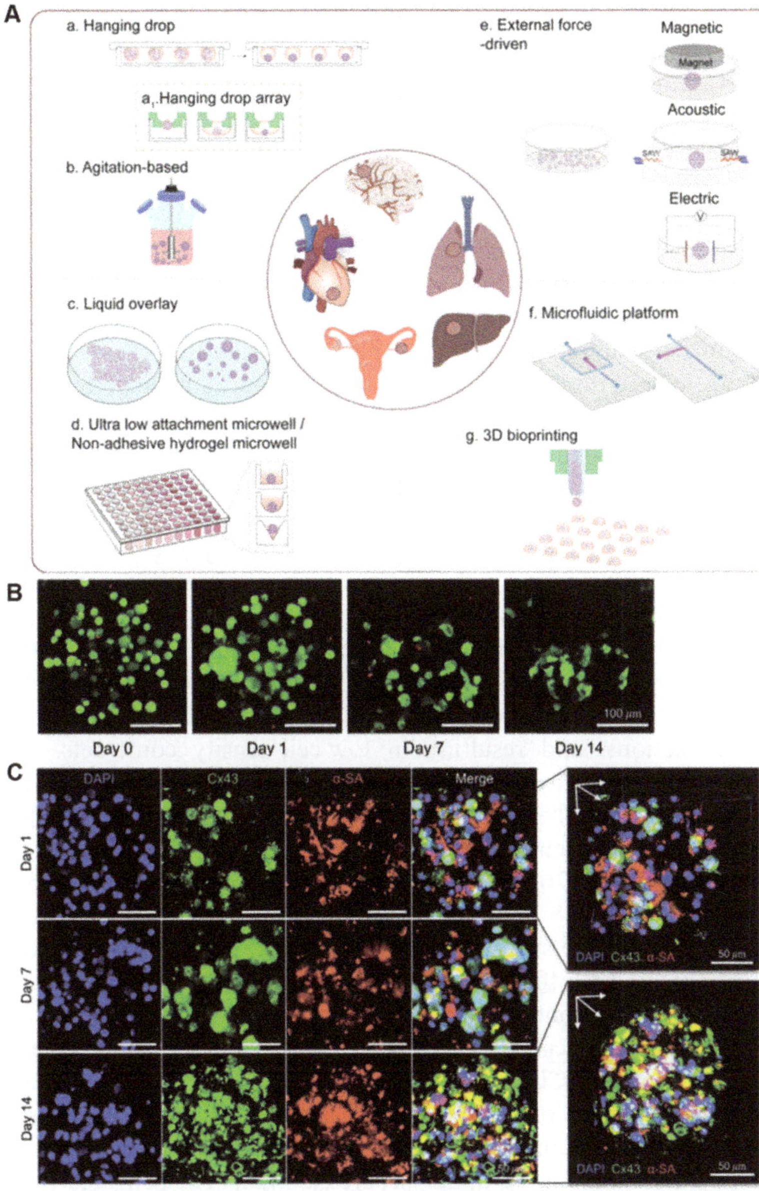

Figure 3.1. Overview of spheroid-utilized 3D bioengineering techniques. (A) Various methods for generating spheroids are suggested; reproduced with permission from reference [19] CC BY 4.0. (B) Example of 3D bioprinted human induced pluripotent stem-cell-derived cardiomyocyte (hiPSC-CM) spheroid. The viability of the hiPSC-CM spheroid was sustained for 14 days, and the evidence was validated by the Live (green)/Dead (red) assay; reproduced with permission from reference [24]. (C) Immunofluorescence staining of connexin 43 (green) and α-SA (red) on days 1, 7, and 14 with 4′,6-diamidino-2-phenylindole (blue) from hiPSC-CM spheroids; reproduced with permission from reference [24] John Wiley & Sons. Copyright 2021 Wiley-VCH GmbH.

three different cell types: neuroblastoma (SK-N-BE(2)), non-small cell lung cancer (H460), and glioblastoma (U87vIII) cells [20]. Three-dimensional (3D) multicellular spheroids were embedded inside a hydrogel matrix with precise size and cell number control. The intra-experimental variability in the coefficient of variation of the embedded spheroid diameter was between 4.2% and 8.7% [20]. The spheroids of human iPSC-derived cardiomyocytes (hiPSC-CMs) offer a myocardial environment where the cells can interact with their surroundings on a 3D level, representing the *in vivo* maturation of adult cardiomyocytes [21–23]. To obtain hiPSC-CMs, Kang *et al* differentiated iPSCs into cardiomyocytes for 16 days and printed spheroidal microtissues containing hiPSC-CMs [24]. The 3D-printed hiPSC-CM spheroids exhibited diameters of up to 200 μm. The encapsulated cells were uniformly distributed throughout the entire volume of the spheroids immediately after printing and matured over the culture period (figure 3.1(B)) [24]. Moreover, the distribution and expression of a gap junction protein, connexin 43, and the actin filament crosslinking protein, α-SA, were successfully enhanced on day 14 after the initial printing (figure 3.1(C)) [24]. Hence, hiPSC-CM spheroids successfully created a continuous cellular network by demonstrating the capacity of intercellular signaling for cardiac development.

The 3D multicellular tumor spheroids can better recapitulate actual 3D tumor behaviors and microenvironments at the phenotypic and genotypic levels to emulate the complexities of living cancer tissues [25]. However, previous studies were predominantly designed to process cancer cells embedded within bioinks, limiting cell-to-cell interactions, and resulting in low-cell-density constructs. This issue motivated the development of an advanced *in vitro* 3D cancer–vascular platform using 3D hypoxic tumor spheroids (metastatic cancer unit (MCU)) and a perfusable vascular endothelium system (VES) to precisely mimic tumor progression and metastasis (figure 3.2(A)) [26, 27]. Following the printing strategy, a tumor with a high cellular density (>108 cells/ml) was directly printed in the form of a 3D spheroid, and the vessel-like structure was finally fabricated in 0.5% of a skin-derived dECM bioink-specific bath (figure 3.2(B)) [26]. Consequently, cancer–vascular interactions were defined by controlling the distance between the MCUs and VES to investigate metastasis-associated changes in the adjacent and distal regions (figure 3.2(C)) [26]. The MCUs proximal to the vessel showed enhanced cancer cell invasion from the surface of the MCUs to the VES via sprouting mechanisms (figure 3.2(D)) [26]. The established tumors can activate endothelial cells via inflammatory cytokine signaling during tumor progression [28]. The activated endothelium can recruit the circulating monocyte, thus causing tissue inflammation in the tumor microenvironment (TME); the secretion of tumor necrosis factor-alpha (TNF-α) was significantly enhanced in the proximal group (76.72 ± 3.1 pg ml^{-1}) over that in the distal group (14.15 ± 2.2 pg ml^{-1}) (figure 3.2(E)) [26]. Further, the expressions of monocyte chemoattractant transcripts (colony-stimulating factor 1 [CSF1] and monocyte chemoattractant protein 1 [MCP1] were enhanced in proximal MCUs and were observed to be greater than (2.5- and 1.6-fold, respectively) the enhancements observed in the distal conditions while also showing the recruitment of augmented monocytes (THP-1) in proximal MCUs (figure 3.2(F)) [26]. Overall, these observations suggest

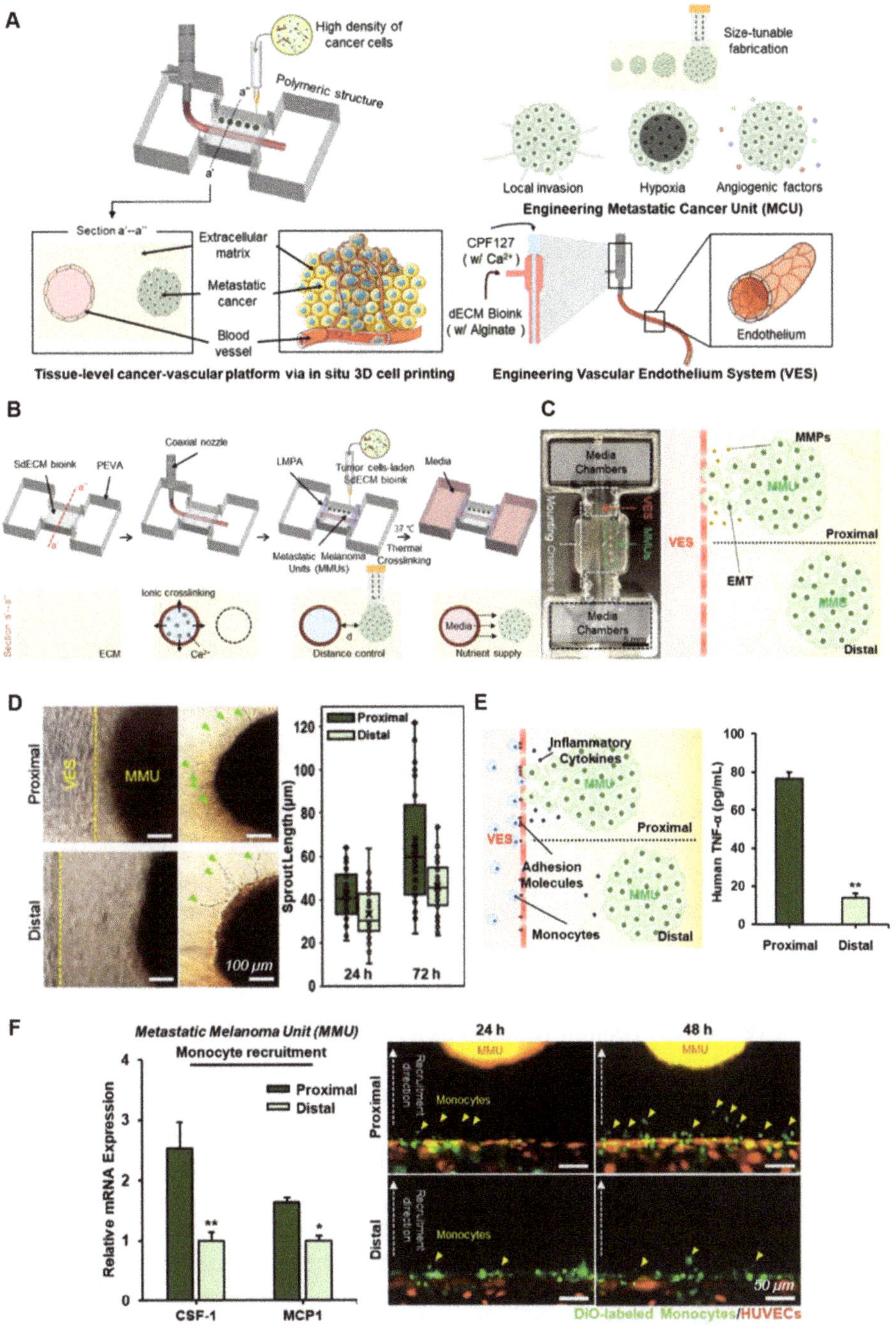

Figure 3.2. Schematic diagram of the utilization of spheroids for the fabrication of a tissue-level cancer–vascular platform and the proposed mechanism. (A) MCUs present with invasiveness, hypoxia, and angiogenic factor secretion. Adjacent perfusable VES was also printed using *in situ* coaxial cell printing. (B) 3D printing processes to fabricate MCUs and VES in a single *in vitro* platform. (C) Representative images

showing distance control of MCUs (proximal or distal to VES). (D) Quantification analysis of sprouting length of MCUs that are proximal and distal to VES. (E) Monocyte recruitment induced inflammatory tumor necrosis factor-alpha (TNF-α) secretion by MCUs on day 3. (F) Quantitative reverse transcription polymerase chain reaction analyses results of the monocytes-recruiting genes colony-stimulating factor 1 and monocyte chemoattractant protein 1 expressions in metastatic melanoma units (left); expressions of DiO-labeled THP-1 cells (green; monocytes) within MCUs; All images were reproduced with permission from reference [26] John Wiley & Sons. Copyright 2021 Wiley-VCH GmbH.

that printed cancer spheroids successfully interacted with the VES unit to establish a complex 3D TME *in vitro*.

Moreover, a blood-lymphatic integrated system with heterogeneous melanoma spheroids (BLISH) has been used to fabricate melanoma microenvironments *in vitro* [29]. Deadly cancers, such as cutaneous melanoma, can quickly transmit to distant organs through the bloodstream and lymphatic system owing to their high metastatic properties [30–35]. Cho *et al* employed an in-bath bioprinting process. They developed a blood-lymphatic integrated system (paired with a biomimetic blood vessel [BV] and lymphatic vessel [LV]) that included metastatic melanoma spheroids (figure 3.3(A)) [29]. *In vitro*, the 3D BV model was coaxially printed with human dermal microvascular endothelial cells, encapsulating a vascular-tissue-derived dECM (VdECM) bioink. At the same time, the LV comprises human-dermal-lymphatic-endothelial-cells-encapsulated VdECM bioink. Moreover, melanoma spheroids were precisely positioned between the BV and LV. Using an *in vitro* 3D BLISH model, Cho *et al* successfully recapitulated the key events of invasive melanoma; melanoma spheroids relentlessly invaded the surrounding VdECM matrix and further adhered to the endothelia of BVs and LVs, while anticancer drugs (emurafenib and pictilsib) significantly decreased the sprouts released from melanoid spheroids (figure 3.3(B)) [29]. In conclusion, using spheroids to construct functional *in vitro* 3D-printed models can create mature native-like microtissues, thereby improving our understanding of cancer progression and the translatability of potential cancer therapeutics.

3.5 Organoids

Organoids have recently been introduced as a novel source for engineering in *in vitro* models using 3D bioprinting. Organoids are developed from pluripotent stem cells (PSCs) or adult stem cells (figure 3.4) [36] and possess key characteristics of their organ counterparts; thus, they can mimic the biological and developmental processes of organs within a 3D *in vitro* environment [37]. Therefore, organoids have promising applications in drug screening, disease modeling, and tissue/organ regeneration. However, while handling organoids, maintaining affordable sizes, vascularization, reproducibility, and precise architecture in time and space are still enormous challenges. Nevertheless, the combination of organoids and bioprinting techniques has overcome these obstacles and has recently yielded organoid-based constructs with improved biological and physiological functions.

To rebuild the components of the human heart, Lee *et al* used a complex collagen scaffold as a freely embeddable suspension hydrogel for printing heart organoids. After combining magnetic resonance imaging results of coronary arteries and 3D

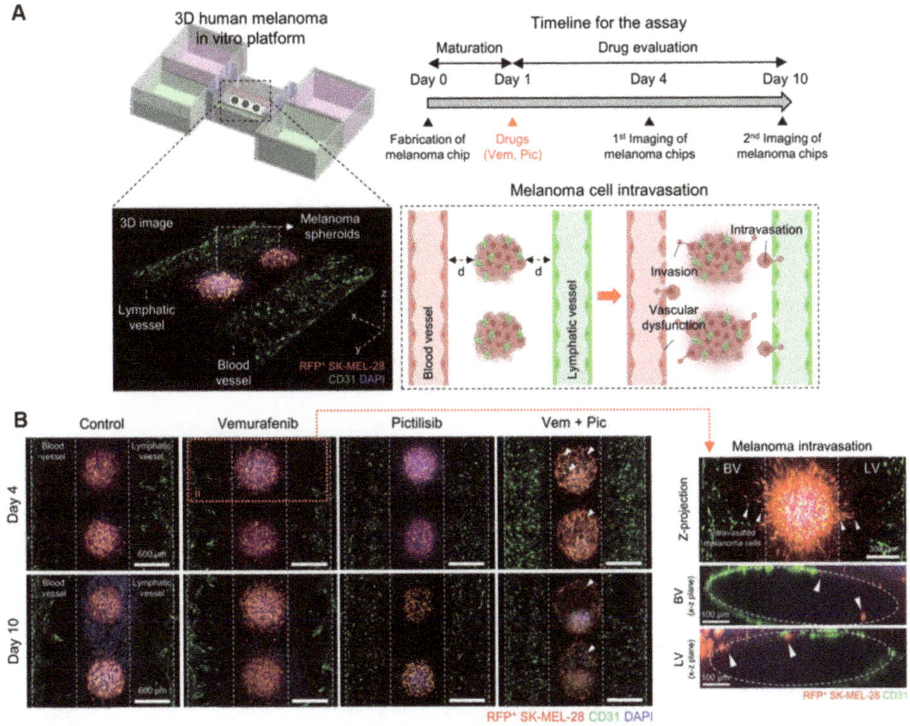

Figure 3.3. Developed 3D human melanoma *in vitro* platform comprises melanoma spheroids, BVs, and LVs. (A) Developed 3D human melanoma *in vitro* platform. The melanoma spheroids, including melanoma cells, were designed to migrate to the adjacent BVs and LVs. (B) Representative 3D confocal images of the *in vitro* 3D melanoma platform. The platform was treated with 5 μM vemurafenib, 5 μM pictilisib, or their combination. The magnified image on the right illustrates the transendothelial migration of SK-MEL-28 spheroids (red; malignant melanoma cell line from the American Type Culture Collection). Melanoma spheroids also exhibit a distorted morphology after drug administration (in the vemurafenib+pictilisib-treated group [white arrow]). Reproduced with permission from reference [29] CC BY 4.0.

images of the heart, they achieved delicate *in vitro* heart structures at different structural scales, from capillaries to the entire heart organ. High-resolution printing of heart organoids also showed systolic function [36, 38]. Lawlor *et al* applied extrusion-based 3D cellular bioprinting to deliver a high-throughput generation of kidney organoids with highly reproducible cell numbers and viability (figure 3.5) [39]. To fabricate multiscale heterogeneous liver tissues and create 3D bioprinted hepato-organoids, Yang *et al* used a mixture of hepatocyte suspensions (1×10^6 HepaRG cells) in 4% sodium alginate-added bioink [40]. HepaRG cells were printed, coated on a culture dish, and matured to build the final liver organoids [40]. Three-dimensionally printed liver organoids formed clusters and achieved liver functions such as albumin secretion and glycogen storage after seven days of differentiation [40].

Moreover, tissue-specific organoids are derived from human PSCs (hPSCs) for *in vitro* recapitulation of the elements of embryonic development. However, they are

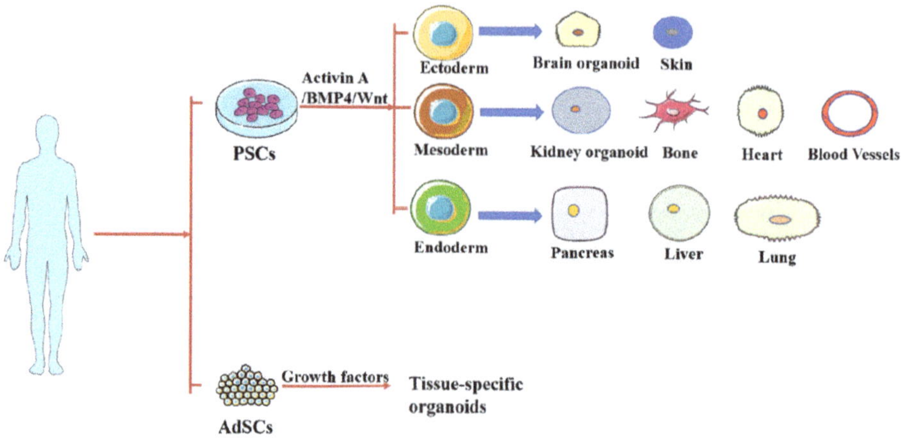

Figure 3.4. Schematic illustration of PSC- and adult stem cell (AdSC)-derived organoids. PSC-derived organoids pass through the endoderm, mesoderm, or ectoderm and are further induced, matured, and differentiated to particular organs after getting specific growth signals. Conversely, AdSC-derived organoids require the segregation of tissue-specific stem cell populations and are further engendered in combination with particular tissue development components; reproduced with permission from reference [36] CC BY 4.0.

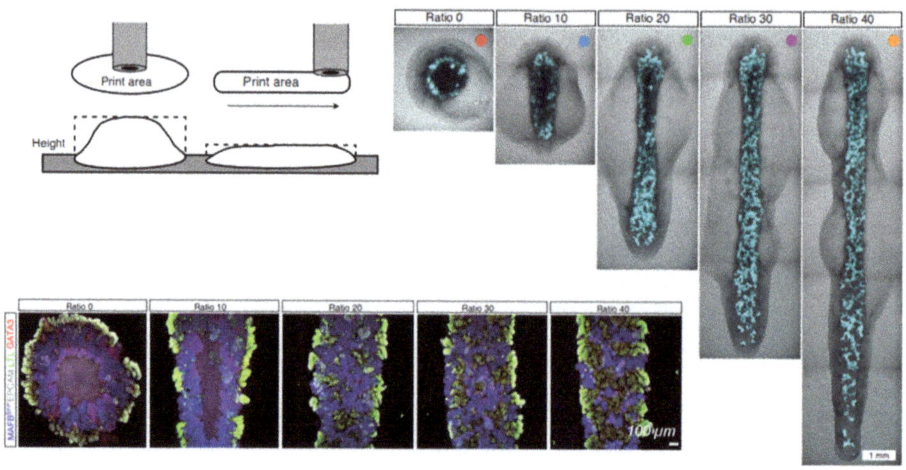

Figure 3.5. Use of extrusion bioprinting to print organoids and alter the organoid conformation/differentiation. Use of extrusion bioprinting to alter kidney organoid conformation. Immunofluorescence of representative bioprinted kidney organoids with various conformations. MAF bZIP transcription factor B gene mTagBFP2 allows the visualization of glomeruli (endogenous blue), epithelial cell adhesion molecule shows the epithelium (gray), lotus tetragonolobus lectin was used to identify the proximal tubule (green), and connecting segment/collecting ducts were marked by GATA binding protein 3 (red); reproduced with permission from reference [39], copyright (2021), with permission from Springer Nature.

not intrinsically vascularized, significantly challenging their sustained growth and the understanding of the role of the vasculature in fate specification and morphogenesis. Salmon *et al* developed an hPSC-based approach to generate organoids that spatially interact with vascular cells (figure 3.6(A)) [41]. The spatial interaction

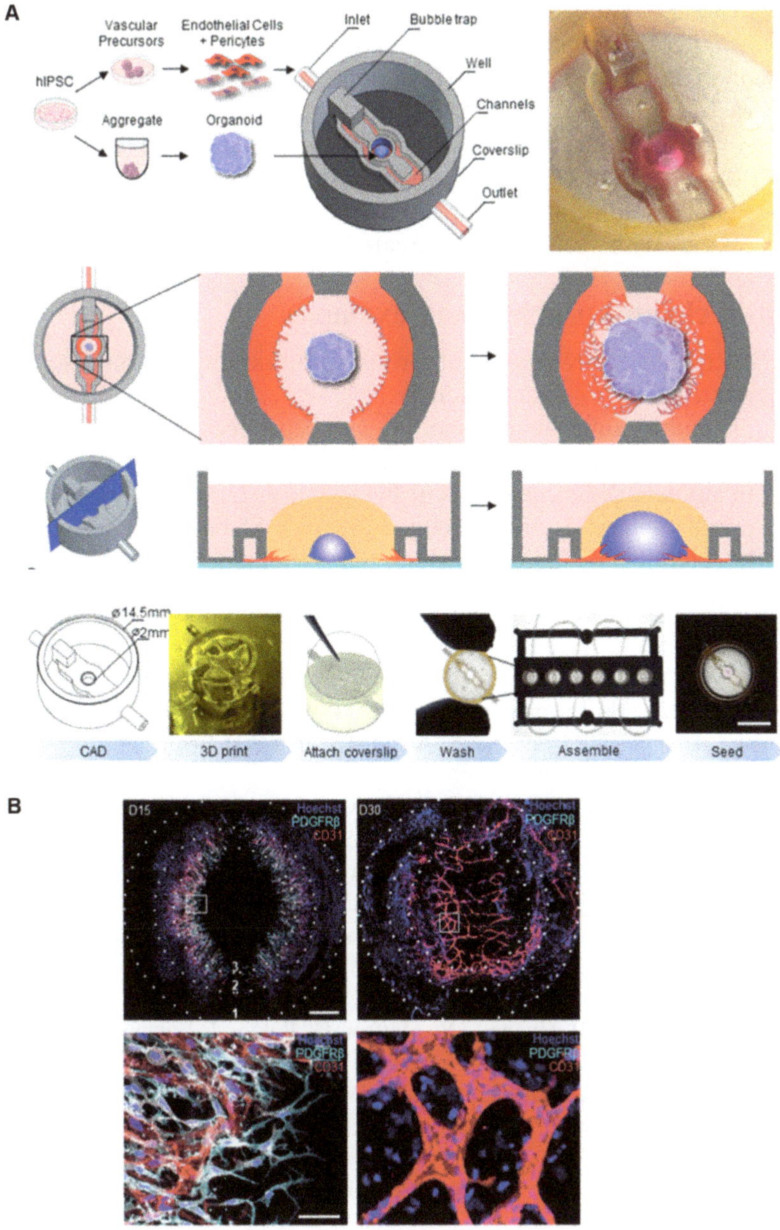

Figure 3.6. Three-dimensionally printed microfluidic platform for vascularized organoid cultures on the chip. (A) Biofabrication of microfluidic chips. The fabrication design was generated in computer-aided design software, and 3D printing was conducted using a FormLabs2 consumer-grade printer. After the seeding of human PSCs, the cells were differentiated into vascular cells or early neural organoids in a suspension on the 3D-printed microfluidic chip. (B) Angiogenic sprouting (CD31-positive vascular networks (red)) was also induced in a vascularized organoid on the chip; reproduced from [41] with permission of The Royal Society of Chemistry.

between the organoid and the vasculature allowed 'on-chip hPSC-derived pericytes and endothelial cells sprout' on day 10, and the self-assembled vascular networks were evident on day 30 (figure 3.6(B)) [41]. In this case, the *in vitro* 3D printing-based platform was designed to be compatible with any organoid system and was also significantly cost-effective for inducing the vascularization of any tissue-specific organoids. In the future, combining organoids and 3D bioprinting will open new avenues for understanding and manipulating the co-development strategies of tissue-specific organoids with vasculature to create highly qualified engineered tissues.

3.6 End-of chapter problem and examples

Q1. Describe the advantages of printing multicellular tumor spheroids for engineering *in vitro* cancer models.

A. 3D multicellular tumor spheroids can better recapitulate actual 3D tumor behaviors and microenvironments at the phenotypic and genotypic levels to emulate the complexities of living cancer tissues. Moreover, when 3D-printed spheroids are embedded in a dECM bath, further cell-to-matrix interactions, including invasion, matrix remodeling, and angiogenesis of cancer spheroids, can be recapitulated.

References

[1] Benam K H *et al* 2015 Engineered *in vitro* disease models *Annu. Rev. Pathol.* **10** 195–262

[2] LeCluyse E L, Bullock P L, Parkinson A and Hochman J H 1996 Cultured rat hepatocytes *Pharm. Biotechnol.* **8** 121–59

[3] Griffith L G, Wu B, Cima M J, Powers M J, Chaignaud B and Vacanti J P 1997 *In vitro* organogenesis of liver tissue *Ann. N. Y. Acad. Sci.* **831** 382–97

[4] Singh N K, Han W, Nam S A, Kim J W, Kim J Y, Kim Y K and Cho D W 2020 Three-dimensional cell-printing of advanced renal tubular tissue analogue *Biomaterials* **232** 119734

[5] Singh N K, Kim J Y, Lee J Y, Lee H, Gao G, Jang J, Kim Y K and Cho D W 2023 Coaxial cell printing of a human glomerular model: an *in vitro* glomerular filtration barrier and its pathophysiology *Biofabrication* **15** 024101

[6] Ong C S, Yesantharao P, Huang C Y, Mattson G, Boktor J, Fukunishi T, Zhang H and Hibino N 2018 3D bioprinting using stem cells *Pediatr. Res.* **83** 223–31

[7] Pati F, Jang J, Ha D H, Won Kim S, Rhie J W, Shim J H, Kim D H and Cho D W 2014 Printing three-dimensional tissue analogues with decellularized extracellular matrix bioink *Nat. Commun.* **5** 3935

[8] Shao G B, Hai R H and Sun C 2020 3D printing customized optical lens in minutes *Adv. Opt. Mater.* **8** 1901646

[9] Gao G *et al* 2017 Tissue engineered bio-blood-vessels constructed using a tissue-specific bioink and 3D coaxial cell printing technique: a novel therapy for ischemic disease *Adv. Funct. Mater.* **27** 1700798

[10] Yi H G *et al* 2019 A bioprinted human-glioblastoma-on-a-chip for the identification of patient-specific responses to chemoradiotherapy *Nat. Biomed. Eng.* **3** 509–19

[11] Das S, Kim S W, Choi Y J, Lee S, Lee S H, Kong J S, Park H J, Cho D W and Jang J 2019 Decellularized extracellular matrix bioinks and the external stimuli to enhance cardiac tissue development *in vitro Acta Biomater.* **95** 188–200

[12] Glicklis R, Merchuk J C and Cohen S 2004 Modeling mass transfer in hepatocyte spheroids via cell viability, spheroid size, and hepatocellular functions *Biotechnol. Bioeng.* **86** 672–80
[13] Takayama K, Nagamoto Y, Mimura N, Tashiro K, Sakurai F, Tachibana M, Hayakawa T, Kawabata K and Mizuguchi H 2013 Long-term self-renewal of human ES/iPS-derived hepatoblast-like cells on human laminin 111-coated dishes *Stem Cell Rep.* **1** 322–35
[14] Mao S, Pang Y, Liu T, Shao Y, He J, Yang H, Mao Y and Sun W 2020 Bioprinting of *in vitro* tumor models for personalized cancer treatment: a review *Biofabrication* **12** 042001
[15] Urciuolo F, Imparato G, Totaro A and Netti P A 2013 Building a tissue *in vitro* from the bottom up: implications in regenerative medicine *Methodist Debakey Cardiovasc. J.* **9** 213–7
[16] Laschke M W and Menger M D 2017 Life is 3D: boosting spheroid function for tissue engineering *Trends Biotechnol.* **35** 133–44
[17] Cui X, Hartanto Y and Zhang H 2017 Advances in multicellular spheroids formation *J. R. Soc. Interface* **14** 20160877
[18] Edmondson R, Broglie J J, Adcock A F and Yang L J 2014 Three-dimensional cell culture systems and their applications in drug discovery and cell-based biosensors *Assay Drug Dev. Tech.* **12** 207–18
[19] Zhuang P, Chiang Y H, Fernanda M S and He M 2021 Using spheroids as building blocks towards 3D bioprinting of tumor microenvironment *Int. J. Bioprint.* **7** 444
[20] Utama R H *et al* 2020 A 3D bioprinter specifically designed for the high-throughput production of matrix-embedded multicellular spheroids *Iscience* **23** 101621
[21] Yan Y W, Bejoy J, Xia J F, Griffin K, Guan J J and Li Y 2019 Cell population balance of cardiovascular spheroids derived from human induced pluripotent stem cells *Sci. Rep.* **9** 1295
[22] Mattapally S, Zhu W, Fast V G, Gao L, Worley C, Kannappan R, Borovjagin A V and Zhang J 2018 Spheroids of cardiomyocytes derived from human-induced pluripotent stem cells improve recovery from myocardial injury in mice *Am. J. Physiol. Heart. Circ. Physiol.* **315** H327–39
[23] Beauchamp P, Jackson C B, Ozhathil L C, Agarkova I, Galindo C L, Sawyer D B, Suter T M and Zuppinger C 2020 3D co-culture of hiPSC-derived cardiomyocytes with cardiac fibroblasts improves tissue-like features of cardiac spheroids *Front. Mol. Biosci.* **7** 14
[24] Kang B, Park Y, Hwang D G, Kim D, Yong U, Lim K S and Jang J 2021 Facile bioprinting process for fabricating size-controllable functional microtissues using light-activated decellularized extracellular matrix-based bioinks *Adv. Mater. Technol.* **7** 2100947
[25] Amaral R L F, Miranda M, Marcato P D and Swiech K 2017 Comparative analysis of 3D bladder tumor spheroids obtained by forced floating and hanging drop methods for drug screening *Front. Physiol.* **8** 605
[26] Kim B S, Cho W W, Gao G, Ahn M, Kim J and Cho D W 2021 Construction of tissue-level cancer-vascular model with high-precision position control via *in situ* 3D cell printing *Small Methods* **5** e2100072
[27] Osaki T, Uzel S G M and Kamm R D 2018 Microphysiological 3D model of amyotrophic lateral sclerosis (ALS) from human iPS-derived muscle cells and optogenetic motor neurons *Sci. Adv.* **4** eaat5847
[28] Klein D 2018 The tumor vascular endothelium as decision maker in cancer therapy *Front. Oncol.* **8** 367
[29] Cho W W, Ahn M, Kim B S and Cho D W 2022 Blood-lymphatic integrated system with heterogeneous melanoma spheroids via in-bath three-dimensional bioprinting for modelling of combinational targeted therapy *Adv. Sci. (Weinh)* **9** e2202093

[30] Ruiter D, Bogenrieder T, Elder D and Herlyn M 2002 Melanoma-stroma interactions: structural and functional aspects *Lancet Oncol.* **3** 35–43

[31] Labrousse A L, Ntayi C, Hornebeck W and Bernard P 2004 Stromal reaction in cutaneous melanoma *Crit. Rev. Oncol. Hemat.* **49** 269–75

[32] Karaman S and Detmar M 2014 Mechanisms of lymphatic metastasis *J. Clin. Invest.* **124** 922–8

[33] Alitalo A and Detmar M 2012 Interaction of tumor cells and lymphatic vessels in cancer progression *Oncogene* **31** 4499–508

[34] Ubellacker J M *et al* 2020 Lymph protects metastasizing melanoma cells from ferroptosis *Nature* **585** 113

[35] Morton D L *et al* 2014 Final trial report of sentinel-node biopsy versus nodal observation in melanoma *New Engl. J. Med.* **370** 599–609

[36] Ren Y *et al* 2021 Developments and opportunities for 3D bioprinted organoids *Int. J. Bioprint.* **7** 364

[37] Fatehullah A, Tan S H and Barker N 2016 Organoids as an *in vitro* model of human development and disease *Nat. Cell Biol.* **18** 246–54

[38] Lee A, Hudson A R, Shiwarski D J, Tashman J W, Hinton T J, Yerneni S, Bliley J M, Campbell P G and Feinberg A W 2019 3D bioprinting of collagen to rebuild components of the human heart *Science* **365** 482–7

[39] Lawlor K T *et al* 2021 Cellular extrusion bioprinting improves kidney organoid reproducibility and conformation *Nat. Mater.* **20** 260–71

[40] Yang H *et al* 2021 Three-dimensional bioprinted hepatorganoids prolong survival of mice with liver failure *Gut* **70** 567–74

[41] Salmon I, Grebenyuk S, Abdel Fattah A R, Rustandi G, Pilkington T, Verfaillie C and Ranga A 2022 Engineering neurovascular organoids with 3D printed microfluidic chips *Lab Chip.* **22** 1615–29

IOP Publishing

Organ Printing (Second Edition)

Jinah Jang, Suhun Chae, Jungbin Yoon, Hyeonji Kim and Wonbin Park

Chapter 4

Biomaterials

In organ printing, various 3D-printable biomaterials are used, depending on the characteristics of the target organs/tissues. Through the years, researchers have investigated the mechanical, rheological, and biochemical properties of various materials. Biomaterials are primarily categorized as synthetic polymers and bioinks. Synthetic biocompatible polymers are used when higher mechanical properties are required; bioinks are biocompatible hydrogels that encapsulate cells, thereby protecting them and providing bioactive cues. In this chapter, we introduce synthetic polymers and bioinks.

4.1 Synthetic polymers

Frameworks physically support 3D-printed tissues/organs. They provide handling grips for *in vivo* implants and retain the various shapes of each batch in *in vitro* models. Synthetic polymers have contributed to the construction of 3D frameworks owing to their controllable properties, good printability without clogging, and flexible versatility under each printing condition. Polycaprolactone (PCL), poly-lactic-co-glycolic acid (PLGA), pluronic acid, polydimethylsiloxane (PDMS), poly (ethylene glycol) (PEG), polyvinyl alcohol (PVA), and their derivatives can provide not only physical and mechanical support to 3D-bioprinted constructs, but also exhibit minimal influence on the cells or cellular behaviors based on their biocompatibility.

4.1.1 Polycaprolactone

PCL is a US Food and Drug Administration (FDA)-approved thermoplastic semi-crystalline polyester that offers advantageous features such as stiffness, biocompatibility, and viscoelasticity [1]. It is preferred for heating-based 3D printing (i.e., fused deposition modeling (FDM)), as the melting temperature of PCL is 55 °C–60 °C [2]. It is widely used as a drug delivery carrier in sutures and as a scaffold for tissue repair because of its long-term stability and slow biodegradability [3]. Generally, it is

doi:10.1088/978-0-7503-5122-5ch4

stable for a period of six months, with a biological half-life of three years. However, because PCL is hydrophobic, cells hardly attach to its surface, resulting in low bioactivity. Recently, improvements in PCL have been proposed to enhance its bioactivity through surface functionalization or chemical modification.

4.1.2 Polylactic-co-glycolic acid

PLGA is a polyester copolymer of hydrophobic lactic acid (LA) and hydrophilic glycolic acid (GA), and varying ratios of LA and GA are used to regulate the biodegradable and hydrophilic properties [4, 5]. The major advantage of copolymers with different ratios of LA and GA is that they have been partially approved by the FDA for use in humans. PLGAs have been investigated in a wide range of biomedical applications, especially for bone regeneration, because their mechanical features are similar to those of human calcareous bone and they are osteoconductive [4]. However, their acidic degradation byproducts and poor mechanical stiffness should be considered. Certain studies have attempted to overcome these limitations by mixing them with PCL, resulting in a decrease in the fracturing and inflammatory reactions of the broken debris.

4.1.3 Pluronic acid

Pluronic acid (poloxamer) is a block copolymer composed of one hydrophobic poly (propylene oxide) (PPO) block and two hydrophilic poly (ethylene oxide) (PEO) blocks, configured in the form of PEO-PPO-PEO [6–8]. Pluronics remain fluid at room temperature and become viscous around normal body temperature. These thermosensitive features are reversible and can be controlled by regulating their concentrations and structures, such as the PPO/PEO ratio and total polymer chain length. They are used as drug/cell carriers, wound dressings, and sacrificial molds. In particular, pluronic F127 exhibits shear-thinning behavior with good shear recovery, which enhances the accuracy of bioprinting. However, pluronics have adverse effects on cell viability during long-term *in vitro* culture. To overcome these limitations, recent studies have reported strategies using chemical modifications based on hydroxyl moieties or blending with cell-familiar hydrogels.

4.1.4 Polydimethylsiloxane

PDMS is a silicone-based organic compound that has been extensively used for engineering of *in vitro* tissue/organ models and in biological devices [9–12]. It is elastomeric, biocompatible, transparent, gas-permeable, and nonflammable. As cured PDMS shows hydrophobic features and high flexibility in the solid state, it is used in the construction of microstructures of transparent devices. Micropatterned or microscale molds can be constructed via soft lithography using PDMS. Several studies have demonstrated that the superior flexibility of PDMS leads to successful construction of microscale channels for significantly small amounts of fluidic flow. With these advantages, soft lithography using PDMS has evolved to fabricate microfluidic or *in vitro* tissue/organ models with precise control of fluids and localization of specific cells at the desired position. Moreover, because PDMS is hydrophobic and has poor cellular attachment, some attempts have been made to modify its surface, such as treatment with charged biomolecules (i.e., collagen and fibronectin).

4.1.5 Poly(ethylene glycol)

PEG is a hydrophilic polymer with a linear or branched structure tailed by an asymmetric or dissymmetric hydroxyl ion [7, 13]. Because of its high tunability, affinity for biomolecules, and resistance to protein adsorption, it is predominantly used in drug delivery systems. In extrusion-based printing, PEG has been used as a sacrificial material for complex and hollow-shaped frameworks owing to its water solubility. To improve cellular interactions, PEG has been conjugated with biomimetic ligands including peptide sequences, proteins, and drugs. Modified or conjugated PEG can then be used for cell encapsulation. The modified PEG offers a cell adhesion site, enhances protein adsorption and covalent coupling with cell-adhesive peptide sequences, and improves mechanical strength.

4.1.6 Polyvinyl alcohol

PVA is a semi-crystalline polymer containing vinyl alcohol and acetate [7, 14, 15]. It is water-soluble, biocompatible, and biodegradable and is predominantly used in FDM- and selective laser sintering (SLS)-based printing techniques. The tensile properties of PVA are similar to those of the human articular cartilage; therefore, it is widely used in numerous load-bearing treatments. PVA is also used in pharmaceutical applications owing to its hydrophilicity and chemical stability under extreme pH and temperature conditions. Dosage forms can be controlled via 3D printing technologies, resulting in different drug release profiles.

4.2 Bioinks

A bioink is a cell-laden hydrogel. Chapter 3 describes the cells used for organ printing. Therefore, in this chapter, we introduce hydrogels as bioinks. Hydrogels provide a cell-friendly matrix to recapitulate native extracellular matrix (ECM) microenvironments because of their tunable physical properties, biodegradability, and bioactivity. Hydrogels that are used as bioinks must satisfy the following requirements: (1) must flow under pressure during the 3D printing process, (2) must display quick gelation kinetics, and (3) must sustain adequate integrity after buildup. In the solution–gelation (sol–gel) transition process, fibrotic molecules in the sol-state hydrogel can be physically or chemically cross-linked by changing the temperature, light source, or ion concentration. The primary advantage of physical cross-linking is the absence of cytotoxic chemical agents. In contrast, chemical cross-linking forms covalent bonds, resulting in superior mechanical properties. The number of hydrogels that are applicable as bioinks is currently limited, and adjusting their physical and chemical properties remains difficult. Natural source-derived hydrogels, such as alginate, collagen, gelatin, cellulose, silk fibroin, matrigel, and dECM, have been widely used as bioinks.

4.2.1 Alginate

Alginate is an anionic block copolymer derived from brown algae [16, 17]. It is a low-cost, biodegradable, and cytocompatible material that can be cross-linked by simple immersion in a $CaCl_2$ solution. Their mechanical properties, including tensile strength, Young's modulus, and elongation, can be controlled by varying the $CaCl_2$ concentration. However, alginate does not provide binding sites for mammalian cells and is therefore bioinert to human cells. Thus, modification of alginates with the addition of arginyl-glycyl-aspartic acid (RGD) or gelatin helped improve cell attachment.

4.2.2 Collagen

Collagen is the most abundant component of mammalian body systems; therefore, it has been used extensively in biomedical applications [18, 19]. The main strength of collagen hydrogels is their ubiquitous nature, which is expected to elicit limited immunogenic responses. However, collagen exhibits poor mechanical properties after thermal cross-linking and a rapid degradation rate. To enhance its mechanical properties, collagen has been combined with chemical cross-linkers or hybridized with other natural molecules (e.g., glycosaminoglycans, tricalcium phosphates) and synthetic polymers (e.g., polyglycerol methacrylate).

4.2.3 Gelatin

Gelatin is a water-soluble protein and a denatured form of collagen produced via hydrolysis [20]. Because gelatin retains the RGD sequence from collagen, it promotes cell adhesion and proliferation. Gelatin possesses most advantages of collagen with a reversal in the sol–gel trends of collagen [21]. Although gelatin dissolves as a colloidal solution at body temperatures, it can form a gel when the temperature drops to <29 °C. This material is limited by its fast degradation and poor mechanical properties; thus, several attempts to improve its properties, including blending with other materials, chemical modifications (e.g., methacrylated gelatin and biomolecule-conjugated gelatin), and use of additive cross-linkers, have been reported.

4.2.4 Cellulose

Cellulose is a biologically derived polysaccharide biopolymer extracted from plants and bacteria (*Acetobacter xylinum* or *Gluconacetobacter xylinus*) [16, 20, 22, 23]. Porous cellulose hydrogels exhibit biocompatibility, biodegradability, hydrophobicity, transparency, desirable mechanical stability, and good cell adhesion properties. Thus, this material can be used as a drug carrier to deliver pharmaceutical agents, contact lenses, and wound healing materials.

4.2.5 Silk fibroin

Silk fibroin is a complex of sericin and fibroin proteins, usually obtained from the silkworm *Bombyx mori* [24, 25]. It has been established as a suitable biomaterial for culturing different cell types, including those of breast cancer, prostate cancer, osteosarcoma, and hepatocellular carcinomas. Among the various types of silk fibroins, silk fibroin hydrogels have good biocompatibility and processability; however, further development is necessary to enhance the tumorigenicity and malignant performance of cancer cells.

4.2.6 Extracellular matrix-based materials

The ECM is a biological network that offers original support to cells and cell–cell communication, providing a physical shape to all biological tissues [26, 27]. It comprises collagen, glycoproteins, proteoglycans, and glycosaminoglycans. Matrigel is derived from a basement membrane composite secreted by Engelbreth–Holm–Swarm mouse sarcoma cells. Therefore, matrigel promotes tumorigenic growth and invasion, and is extensively used for the culture of tumor cells. In contrast, dECM emulates the native composition of the tissue matrix, which is the most desirable material. Decellularization is the process of removing residing cells and retaining the ECM from tissues and organs. The high efficiency of decellularization can provide tissue-specific ECM compositions. As dECM contains a large portion of collagen, it can be solubilized through pepsin-mediated digestion. The solubilized dECM exhibited cross-linking properties at physiologically relevant pH values and temperatures. Moreover, as they recapitulate the native environment of each tissue, dECM hydrogels have promoted cellular activities when compared to single-element-containing hydrogels such as collagen. However, certain limitations in printability have been reported, and attempts to improve their mechanical properties have recently been carried out [28].

4.3 End-of chapter problem and examples

Q. Describe the major requirements of bioinks.

A. Hydrogels must satisfy the following requirements for use as bioinks: (1) to flow under pressure during the 3D printing process (shear-thinning behavior), (2) to display quick gelation kinetics based on physical or chemical cross-linking, and (3) to sustain adequate integrity after 3D printing.

References

[1] Yang X, Wang Y, Zhou Y, Chen J and Wan Q 2021 The application of polycaprolactone in three-dimensional printing scaffolds for bone tissue engineering *Polymers* **13** 2754

[2] She Y, Fan Z, Wang L, Li Y, Sun W, Tang H, Zhang L, Wu L, Zheng H and Chen C 2021 3D printed biomimetic PCL scaffold as framework interspersed with collagen for long segment tracheal replacement *Front. Cell Develop. Biol.* **9** 629796

[3] Mondal D, Griffith M and Venkatraman S S 2016 Polycaprolactone-based biomaterials for tissue engineering and drug delivery: current scenario and challenges *Int. J. Polym. Mater. Polym. Biomater.* **65** 255–65

[4] Sun F, Sun X, Wang H, Li C, Zhao Y, Tian J and Lin Y 2022 Application of 3D-printed, PLGA-based scaffolds in bone tissue engineering *Int. J. Mol. Sci.* **23** 5831

[5] Guo T, Holzberg T R, Lim C G, Gao F, Gargava A, Trachtenberg J E, Mikos A G and Fisher J P 2017 3D printing PLGA: a quantitative examination of the effects of polymer composition and printing parameters on print resolution *Biofabrication* **9** 024101

[6] Müller M, Becher J, Schnabelrauch M and Zenobi-Wong M 2015 Nanostructured Pluronic hydrogels as bioinks for 3D bioprinting *Biofabrication* **7** 035006

[7] Vanaei S, Parizi M, Salemizadehparizi F and Vanaei H 2021 An overview on materials and techniques in 3D bioprinting toward biomedical application *Eng. Regen.* **2** 1–18

[8] Russo E and Villa C 2019 Poloxamer hydrogels for biomedical applications *Pharmaceutics* **11** 671

[9] Ozbolat V, Dey M, Ayan B, Povilianskas A, Demirel M C and Ozbolat I T 2018 3D printing of PDMS improves its mechanical and cell adhesion properties *ACS Biomater. Sci. Eng.* **4** 682–93

[10] Zheng R, Chen Y, Chi H, Qiu H, Xue H and Bai H 2020 3D printing of a polydimethylsiloxane/polytetrafluoroethylene composite elastomer and its application in a triboelectric nanogenerator *ACS Appl. Mater. Interfaces* **12** 57441–9

[11] Venzac B, Deng S, Mahmoud Z, Lenferink A, Costa A, Bray F, Otto C, Rolando C and Le Gac S 2021 PDMS curing inhibition on 3D-printed molds: why? Also, how to avoid it? *Anal. Chem.* **93** 7180–7

[12] Suntornnond R, Tan E Y S, An J and Chua C K 2017 A highly printable and biocompatible hydrogel composite for direct printing of soft and perfusable vasculature-like structures *Sci. Rep.* **7** 1–11

[13] Zhu J 2010 Bioactive modification of poly (ethylene glycol) hydrogels for tissue engineering *Biomaterials* **31** 4639–56

[14] Matijašić G, Gretić M, Vinčić J, Poropat A, Cuculić L and Rahelić T 2019 Design and 3D printing of multi-compartmental PVA capsules for drug delivery *J. Drug Deliv. Sci. Technol.* **52** 677–86

[15] Basa B, Jakab G, Kállai-Szabó N, Borbás B, Fülöp V, Balogh E and Antal I 2021 Evaluation of biodegradable PVA-based 3D printed carriers during dissolution *Materials* **14** 1350

[16] Yi H-G, Kim H, Kwon J, Choi Y-J, Jang J and Cho D-W 2021 Application of 3D bioprinting in the prevention and the therapy for human diseases *Signal Transduct. Target. Ther.* **6** 1–17

[17] Mallakpour S, Azadi E and Hussain C M 2021 State-of-the-art of 3D printing technology of alginate-based hydrogels—an emerging technique for industrial applications *Adv. Colloid Interface Sci.* **293** 102436

[18] Marques C, Diogo G, Pina S, Oliveira J M, Silva T and Reis R 2019 Collagen-based bioinks for hard tissue engineering applications: a comprehensive review *J. Mater. Sci., Mater. Med.* **30** 1–12

[19] Osidak E O, Kozhukhov V I, Osidak M S and Domogatsky S P 2020 Collagen as bioink for bioprinting: a comprehensive review *Int. J. Bioprint.* **6**

[20] Bartolo P, Malshe A, Ferraris E and Koc B 2022 3D bioprinting: materials, processes, and applications *CIRP Ann.* **71** 577–97

[21] Kim H, Jang J-H, Han W, Hwang H-J, Jang J, Kim J Y and Cho D-W 2022 Extracellular matrix-based sticky sealants for scar-free corneal tissue reconstruction *Biomaterials* 121941

[22] Sultan S, Siqueira G, Zimmermann T and Mathew A P 2017 3D printing of nano-cellulosic biomaterials for medical applications *Curr. Opin. Biomed. Eng.* **2** 29–34

[23] Wang Q, Sun J, Yao Q, Ji C, Liu J and Zhu Q 2018 3D printing with cellulose materials *Cellulose* **25** 4275–301
[24] Rodriguez M J, Dixon T A, Cohen E, Huang W, Omenetto F G and Kaplan D L 2018 3D freeform printing of silk fibroin *Acta Biomater.* **71** 379–87
[25] Wang Q, Han G, Yan S and Zhang Q 2019 3D printing of silk fibroin for biomedical applications *Materials* **12** 504
[26] Kim B S, Kim H, Gao G, Jang J and Cho D-W 2017 Decellularized extracellular matrix: a step towards the next generation source for bioink manufacturing *Biofabrication* **9** 034104
[27] Kim B S, Das S, Jang J and Cho D-W 2020 Decellularized extracellular matrix-based bioinks for engineering tissue-and organ-specific microenvironments *Chem. Rev.* **120** 10608–61
[28] Kim H, Kang B, Cui X, Lee S H, Lee K, Cho D W, Hwang W, Woodfield T B, Lim K S and Jang J 2021 Light-activated decellularized extracellular matrix-based bioinks for volumetric tissue analogs at the centimeter scale *Adv. Funct. Mater.* 2011252

IOP Publishing

Organ Printing (Second Edition)

Jinah Jang, Suhun Chae, Jungbin Yoon, Hyeonji Kim and Wonbin Park

Chapter 5

Three-dimensional (3D) bioprinting application for tissue engineering

Organ printing technology has made breakthroughs in the construction of transplantable functional tissue/organ constructs. The 3D bioprinted constructs can replace donor organs, ultimately overcoming organ shortage. Considering orthopedic, cardiac, vascular, and superficial tissues as examples, this chapter delineates the recent advances in several 3D bioprinted tissue/organ substitutes that were validated through *in vivo* trials.

5.1 3D bioprinted orthopedic tissue engineering

Bone contains a hierarchically structured bioceramic composite matrix in which the inorganic (mainly hydroxyapatite) and organic components (primarily type I collagen) are arranged into a well-organized structure that confers the specific mechanical strength of bone. Bone healing represents a mechanobiologically complex process in which osteogenic cells manipulate bone matrix depositions and maintain structural and functional stability [1, 2]. However, an intrinsic limit to its self-healing ability exists depending on the severity of the defect. In humans, critical-sized bone defects larger than 2.5 cm in length do not heal immediately within the lifetime of a patient [3]. Current treatment options, such as bone grafting, have exhibited complications and other drawbacks, including lack of availability, infections, and donor site morbidity; hence, regeneration to counter large bone defects remains a significant ongoing challenge [2, 4]. To circumvent this, 3D bioprinting has been proven to be beneficial for generating customized implants for bone reconstruction. To recapitulate complex organic and inorganic bony micro-environments, 3D bioprinting of cell-laden hydrogel constructs, together with biodegradable polymers and bioceramics, can result in internal porous structures that allow nutrient diffusion. For example, Lee *et al* [5] constructed a 3D cell-laden grid structure using a methacrylated bone decellularized extracellular matrix

doi:10.1088/978-0-7503-5122-5ch5

(dECM) with an alginate bioink, resulting in good biocompatibility and the enhancement of calcium deposition and osteogenic differentiation *in vitro*. Similarly, Kim *et al* [6] developed a 3D porous human adipose stem cells (hASCs)-laden construct for a collagen/bioceramic-based bioink. The reconstitution of a composite microenvironment by introducing type I collagen ink and bioceramic particles promoted efficient proliferation and osteogenesis of encapsulated hASCs in the bioprinted constructs. Kang *et al* [7] created complex cellular contructs that were clinically relevant in terms of size, shape, and structural integrity using a multihead extrusion bioprinting system. Bioprinting of stem cell-laden fibrinogen-based composite bioinks along with biodegradable polymers in integrated patterns ensured mechanical stability, and the incorporation of microchannels facilitated the diffusion of nutrients. Using a predesigned patterning approach, they successfully fabricated human-sized bone constructs with arbitrary shapes. On implantation into a rodent model with calvarial bone defects, the bioprinted constructs showed mature bone formation along with evidence of vascularization without necrosis throughout the construct five months after *in vivo* implantation.

Cartilaginous tissues (e.g., articular cartilage and meniscus) are another major constituent of the skeletal system that exists in the joints between bones to alleviate friction; they exhibit superior lubricating properties and load-bearing capacity. These tissues have a heterogeneous zonal arrangement with a hypocellular, avascular, and aneural nature; thus, their self-repair capacity is extremely low. Cartilage injury is prevalent and often leads to irreversible joint dysfunction (e.g., cartilage degeneration and osteoarthritis), causing unbearable pain and reduced range of motion. Consequently, innovative methods for cartilage engineering and regeneration must be urgently developed. Many attempts have been made to mimic the complex properties of native cartilaginous tissues using 3D bioprinting. For example, Melo *et al* [8] fabricated a cartilage-like tissue construct with spatially controlled mechanical properties using an embedding bioprinting approach. Within the printed construct, a human mesenchymal stem cell (hMSC) spheroid-laden fibrinogen bioink (offering a soft microenvironment to reproduce cartilage matrix formation) was locally positioned in a polyethylene glycol (PEG)/alginate/thrombin hydrogel bath of mechanically robust ECM in the MPa range, which is comparable to that of the native cartilage. In another study, Sun *et al* [9] demonstrated a one-step bioprinting of MSC-laden constructs with a gradient structure and zone-specific biochemical microenvironments. They created a gradient-structured multiphasic scaffold mimicking a four-layered osteochondral tissue for anisotropic osteochondral regeneration (figure 5.1(A)). Dual-growth-factor-releasing MSC-laden hydrogels have been utilized for anisotropic chondrogenic differentiation. To support bioink deposition and overall structural integrity, porous poly(ε-caprolactone) (PCL) frameworks with varying gradient pore sizes (750, 550, 350, and 150 μm; from bottom to top) were fabricated using 3D bioprinting. The gradient structure enabled directional cartilage matrix secretion from the resident MSCs, similar to the arrangement of chondrocytes in native cartilage tissue. The construct was implanted in a rabbit osteochondral defect model; a six-month follow-up analysis indicated that the 3D bioprinted gradient-structured cartilage construct provided a

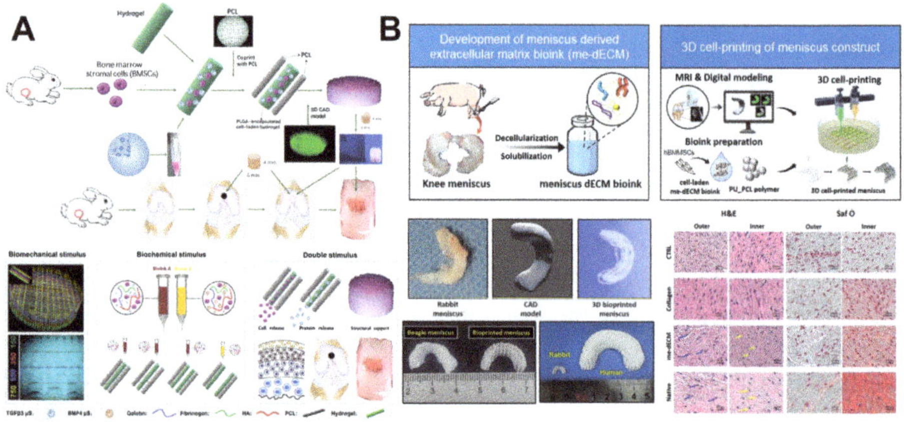

Figure 5.1. 3D bioprinting of cartilage-like constructs. (A) One-step bioprinting of stem cell-laden constructs with gradient structure and zone-specific biochemical microenvironments for articular cartilage regeneration; reproduced with permission from reference [9] CC BY4.0. (B) 3D cell-printing of meniscus construct with meniscus-specific decellularized extracellular matrix (dECM) bioink encapsulating human bone marrow-derived mesenchymal stem cells (hBMSCs) for meniscus regeneration; reproduced with permission from reference [10], copyright (2021), with permission from Elsevier.

mechanically stable environment for spatiotemporal release of cells and bioinstructive proteins, which achieved anisotropic osteochondral regeneration. In meniscal tissue engineering, the meniscus is composed of a fibrocartilage structure within a knee joint, which aids in load bearing and shock absorption. The construction of an intricate zonal organization with robust mechanical properties in the meniscus is challenging. In this case, 3D bioprinting allows for the construction of mechanically strong and anatomically similar structures with high bioactivity. Chae *et al* [10] developed implantable cell-printed meniscal constructs using a mixture of polyurethane and PCL synthetic polymers for mechanical durability, and a stem cell-laden meniscal dECM bioink for improving bioactivity (figure 5.1(B)). Comprehensive *in vivo* evaluations of ectopic mouse and orthotopic rabbit models were performed; the developed bioprinted constructs exhibited prominent biocompatibility and supported neofibrocartilage formation with strong mechanical properties, reminiscent of the native meniscus.

Thus, 3D bioprinting has shown promising potential in the development of biomimitic constructs in combination with cells, biomaterials, and bioactive molecules for orthopedic tissue engineering applications. Notably, 3D bioprinting enables the creation of anatomically accurate scaffolds to promote the regenerative healing of complex orthopedic tissues, presenting a significant translational potential in generating ready-to-implant materials for clinical application.

5.2 3D bioprinted cardiac tissue engineering

The heart is the most vital organ in the body and is responsible for the continuous circulation of blood throughout the body. In consists of various cell types, including fibroblasts, endothelial cells, cardiomyocytes, and smooth muscle cells in a highly compartmentalized manner [11]. Cardiovascular disease remains one of the leading causes of mortality worldwide, and heart transplantation is currently the primary treatment option for end-stage heart failure diseases [12]. However, the general challenges include the lack of available donors and a high risk of immune rejection and surgical complications. 3D bioprinting approaches are promising for engineering cardiac tissues that can replicate the structure of natural myocardial tissues. Among various strategies, stem cell-laden 3D bioprinted cardiac patches provide an alternative and promising solution for the treatment of myocardial infarction (MI). Multiple cell types are useful for bioprinting applications, including induced pluripotent stem cells (iPSCs), MSCs, and embryonic stem cells (ESCs) [13–15], which have cardiac regenerative potential. Jang *et al* [16] reported multicellular and multilayered 3D constructs via the spatial patterning of stem cell sources (human cardiac progenitor cells and MSCs) and pro-angiogenic growth factors to achieve a prevascularized cardiac patch (figure 5.2(A)). A patch with heart dECM bioink improved cell–cell interactions and differentiation capability. Following *in vivo* implantation in a rat MI model, the bioprinted prevascularized patch demonstrated enhanced cardiac function, reduced cardiac hypertrophy and fibrosis, increased stem

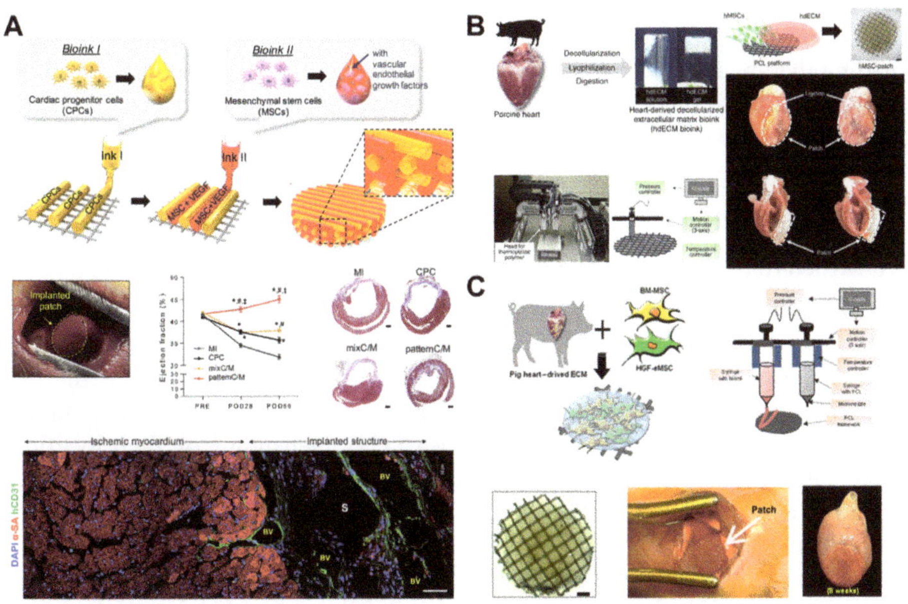

Figure 5.2. 3D bioprinting of stem-laden cardiac patch. (A) 3D prevascularized stem cell patch through spatial patterning of cardiac progenitor/MSCs to enhance the therapeutic efficacy for cardiac repair; reproduced with permission from reference [16], copyright (2017), with permission from Elsevier. (B) Dual stem cell approach of intramyocardially injected hiPSC-CMs and epicardially implanted human MSC-loaded patches to synergistically augment cardiac repair in a rat MI model; reproduced with permission from reference [17] CC BY 4.0. (C) Bioprinted cardiac path with hBMSCs and hepatocyte growth factor–expressing MSCs to enhance the cardiac repair using rat MI model. Reprinted with permission of AAAS from [18] copyright The Authors, some rights reserved; exclusive licensee AAAS. Distributed under a CC BY-NC 4.0 License (http://creativecommons.org/licenses/by-nc/4.0/).

cell migration into the infarcted region, and neo-muscle and capillary formation. Similarly, Park *et al* [17] reported a dual stem cell approach to investigate the synergistic effects of two types of stem cells on cardiac repair (figure 5.2(B)). Specifically, intramyocardially injected human induced pluripotent stem cell-derived cardiomyocytes (hiPSC-CMs) and epicardially implanted hMSC-loaded patches (hMSC-PAs) synergistically improved cardiac function and augmented vascularization post MI. The epicardially implanted hMSC-PA promoted vascular regeneration via prolonged secretion of paracrine signals. More importantly, it considerably enhanced the retention and engraftment of intramyocardially injected hiPSC-CMs, ultimately leading to the restoration of cardiac function. To further improve the therapeutic potential of hMSCs, Park *et al* [18] bioprinted a cardiac path using human bone marrow-derived MSCs (hBMSCs) and genetically modified BMSCs expressing hepatocyte growth factor (HGF-eMSCs) to enhance cardiac repair in a rat MI model (figure 5.2(C)). *In vivo* priming of hBMSCs by prolonged paracrine activity secreted from colocalized HGF-eMSCs in the patch improved vasculogenic potential and high cell viability, resulting in augmented cardioprotection and restored cardiac function in the MI hearts.

Despite promising preclinical outcomes, 3D bioprinting of stem cell-laden cardiac patches is still in its infancy for direct clinical adaptation. Nevertheless, the combination of 3D bioprinting and stem cell technology is evidently beneficial for providing therapeutic and regenerative approaches to overcome ischemic cardiomyopathy. Thus, 3D bioprinted stem cell delivery platforms are a promising means of cardiac repair and regeneration.

5.3 3D bioprinted vascular tissue engineering

5.3.1 Structural, compositional, and mechanical features of blood vessels

The vascular system consists of over 60 000 miles of blood vessels that transport oxygen- and nutrient-rich blood and remove metabolic waste throughout the entire body [19, 20]. Undoubtedly, all organs depend on the performance of the blood vessels for survival. The blood following the vascular network circulates unidirectionally from the heart and returns to the heart [21]. Depending on their location or hemodynamic characteristics, the blood vessels show unique mechanical and physiological features that are imparted by the structure and composition of the vascular wall (figure 5.3).

The vascular wall is composed of three layers: tunica intima, tunica media, and tunica adventitia [22]. Each layer has a typical cellular and biochemical organization. The tunica intima, the innermost layer, consists of aligned endothelial cells. By covering the luminal surface of the blood vessels, endothelial linings tightly regulate the microenvironment of interstitial tissues as a biophysical barrier. The tunica media, that is, the middle layer, comprises smooth muscle cells, elastin, and collagen fibers that provide supportive functions to control the blood flow and pressure by modulating vessel diameter. The tunica adventitia, the outermost layer, is a connective tissue composed of fibroblasts, elastin, and collagen fibers. Based on

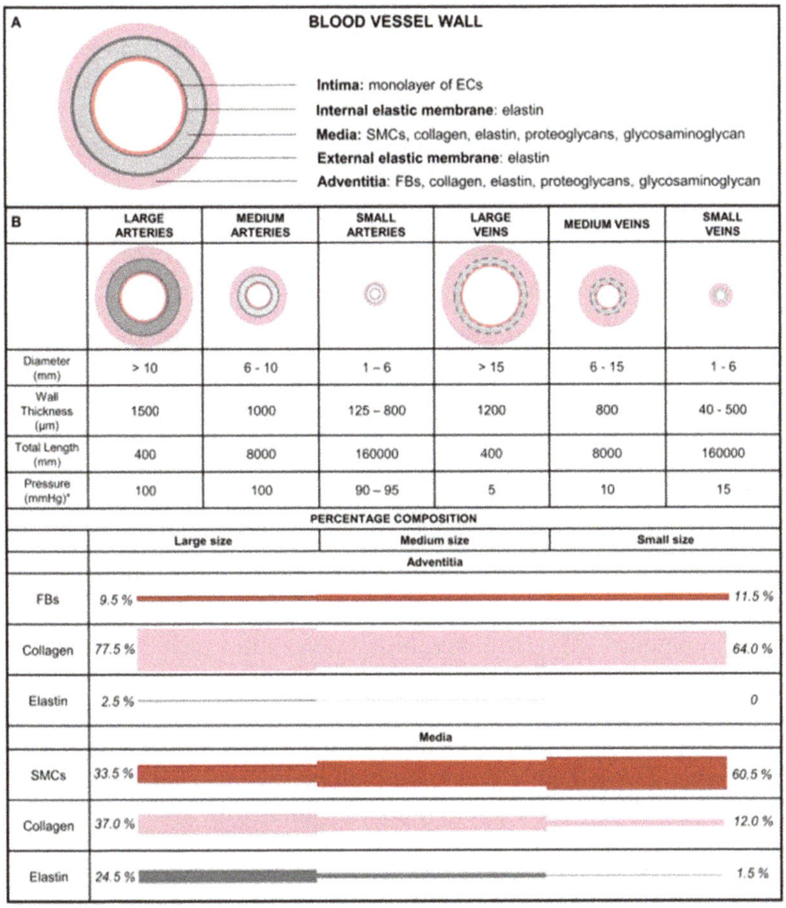

Figure 5.3. Anatomical and functional features of blood vessels. (A) Blood vessel walls generally have three layers: intima, medial, and adventitia. Between each layer, an elastin membrane exists. (B) According to dimensions such as diameter, wall thickness, and composition, the blood vessel can be categorized into three types: arteries, veins, and capillaries. The large vasculatures have higher amount of collagen and elastin, whereas the small vasculatures have higher amount of fibroblasts and smooth muscle cells; reproduced from [22], copyright (2021), with permission from Elsevier.

the wall thickness and proportion of their constituents, the blood vessels are categorized into three main types: arteries, capillaries, and veins.

The arteries are the blood vessels that carry blood away from the heart [23]. Because the heart contracts with high pressure (~120 mmHg) to pump blood to each corner of the body, the connected arteries have thick (<2 mm) and highly elastic walls to withstand the contractile pressure. Narrowing from the heart to distant tissues (25–0.01 mm), the arteries progressively branch and reach the capillaries with small diameters but a large total surface area. The capillaries have the smallest vascular diameter of 5–10 μm. Because capillaries consist of endothelial monolayers with high permeability, molecular exchange can easily occur, nourishing all other tissues by delivering nutrients while removing metabolic byproducts. Capillary pressure differs among tissues (e.g., ~50 mmHg for kidney glomerular capillaries and ~15 mmHg for pulmonary capillaries). After the capillaries merge into veins, oxygen-depleted blood is transported to the heart. The veins also have three layers of walls, but the thickness of the tunica media is less than that of the arteries. Although veins have a relatively low blood pressure (approximately 5–15 mmHg), the blood does not flow backward owing to the existence of venous valves and the surrounding muscular movement. Normally, the tensile strength ranges from 80 to 150 kPa and compressive strength is approximately 10–20 kPa.

5.3.2 3D bioprinting of vascular graft for vascular tissue regeneration

Dysfunction of the vascular system is the leading cause of death globally, with approximately 17.9 million people dying every year because of critical pathological abnormalities such as hypertension and atherosclerosis [24]. The use of autologous arteries or veins is the gold standard for the treatment of diseases; however, this method is accompanied by invasive harvesting and large segmental defects. Currently, damaged blood vessels are being replaced by synthetic prostheses with polyethylene terephthalate or expanded polytetrafluoroethylene, and these synthetic grafts have shown efficient adaptability to large-diameter blood vessels (>6 mm) with long-term patency [25]. However, high failure rates have been reported in the application for small-diameter blood vessels (<5–6 mm), together with a high incidence of thrombosis and stenosis resulting from poor biocompatibility and mismatched biomechanical properties [26]. To overcome these limitations, intensive efforts have been devoted for developing biomimetic vascular grafts. Particularly, biocompatible prostheses should retain endothelialization and possess appropriate mechanical properties such as burst pressure, compliance, and suture retention. This chapter focuses on tissue engineering approaches that use 3D bioprinting technology to construct artificial vascular conduits.

3D bioprinting strategies to recapitulate complex vascular structures have attracted tremendous attention globally because of their high flexibility in using various biomaterials and their fidelity in obtaining precise dimensions with multi-scale applicability. Unique dimensional integrity, including in layers, inner diameters, and wall thicknesses, can be easily achieved using this technology. One strategy involves printing vascular grafts using a scaffold-based method. Szklanny *et al* attempted to build engineered tissue flaps using hierarchical vessel networks. After creating a poly(l-lactide) (PLLA)-poly(lactic-co-glycolic) acid (PLGA) scaffold using a 3D printed mold, endothelial cells were seeded onto the fibrin-coated inner wall [27]. Endothelial cell- and smooth muscle cell-laden recombinant human collagen methacrylate bioinks were printed to generate surrounding vascularized tissues. Physical assembly of the scaffold and vascularized constructs provided a chance to generate a vascular interconnection between the two structures that fully engineered vessel flaps with functional hierarchical vascular networks. Su *et al* used a gelatin/chitosan hybrid solution to fabricate a complex vascular network in heterogeneous porous scaffolds [28]. The stimuli-responsive hydrogels formed networks cued by multiple stimuli, including temperature, sodium sulfate, and sodium

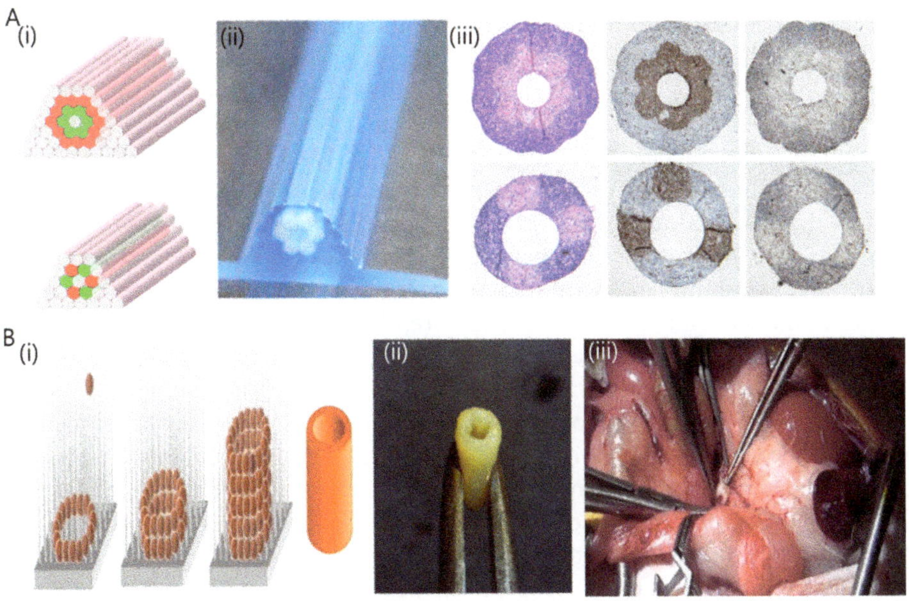

Figure 5.4. 3D bioprinting of scaffold-free vascular tissue. (A) Tubular constructs with multicellular cylinders were fabricated. (i), (ii) Through layer-by-layer deposition process, various types of multicellular cylinders could be assembled. (iii) After three days, mature vascular constructs with structural complexity were generated [29], copyright (2009), with permission from Elsevier. (B) By combining needle-array technology with 3D bioprinting technology, a scaffold-free vascular graft was fabricated with multicellular spheroids. (i) By skewering the spheroids into needle array, tubular structures could be generated. (ii) Image captured after maturation. (iii) Vascular grafts were successfully implanted into infrarenal abdominal aortas of nude rats; reproduced with permission from reference [30] CC BY 4.0.

hydroxide, which generated multifurcated hydrogel tubes. Depending on the sulfate treatment time, mechanical properties, including burst pressure and suture retention strength, increased. The scaffolds provided structural diversity to the constructs used in previous studies. However, the scaffold-based approaches require complicated processes involving multiple steps, such as scaffold fabrication and cell seeding. Moreover, the seeding of endothelial cells to form the endothelium is unstable, and the efficacy of this process depends on multiple factors, including cell density, seeding time, and cellular affinity on the scaffold surface.

The 3D bioprinting technology can also be used to organize cellular strands and aggregates containing endothelial cells to generate vasculatures. During maturation, each patterned structure can be fused to form blood vessel-like constructs. Norotte *et al* printed multicellular spheroids or cylinders under precise diameter control (300–500 μm) and cultured the structure to fabricate hollow cylinders (figure 5.4(A)) [29]. After the fusion of the spheroids, agarose mold was eliminated and multi-layered and bifurcated blood vessels containing various vascular cell types with an outer diameter of 0.9–2.5 mm were successfully fabricated. Conversely, multicellular spheroids composed of endothelial cells, smooth muscle cells, and fibroblasts were manipulated by a robotically controlled fine suction nozzle (outer and inner diameters of 0.45 and 0.23 mm, respectively) and placed into a needle array to form scaffold-free tubular tissue (figure 5.4(B)) [30]. After four days of fusion among the spheroids, the constructs were dynamically cultured under 2–4 ml min^{-1} of media flow. Fully mature vascular grafts exhibited an extensive collagenous ECM and possessed distributed cluster of differentiation (CD) 31-positive cells that were distributed to all parts. Conversely, five days after the implantation of the constructs into the infrarenal abdominal aortas of nude mice, aligned endothelial cells along the lumen could be generated. Although the scaffold-free approach could be achieved using only cells, additional operational procedures were required to generate densely integrated multicellular spheres. Furthermore, the mechanical properties at approximately 939 mN resulted in several limitations regarding the long-term observations.

As an alternative approach, 3D coaxial bioprinting technology, which is a direct printing method for hollow conduits using a coaxial nozzle, was developed. The coaxial nozzle consists of core and shell nozzles, and two different materials can be simultaneously extruded to generate a core/shell filament. The cross-linking of the shell filament and elimination of the core filament allow the direct production of a cylindrical tube. Gao *et al* developed a vascular graft using this technology (figure 5.5(A)) [31]. To introduce a tissue-specific microenvironment, the authors

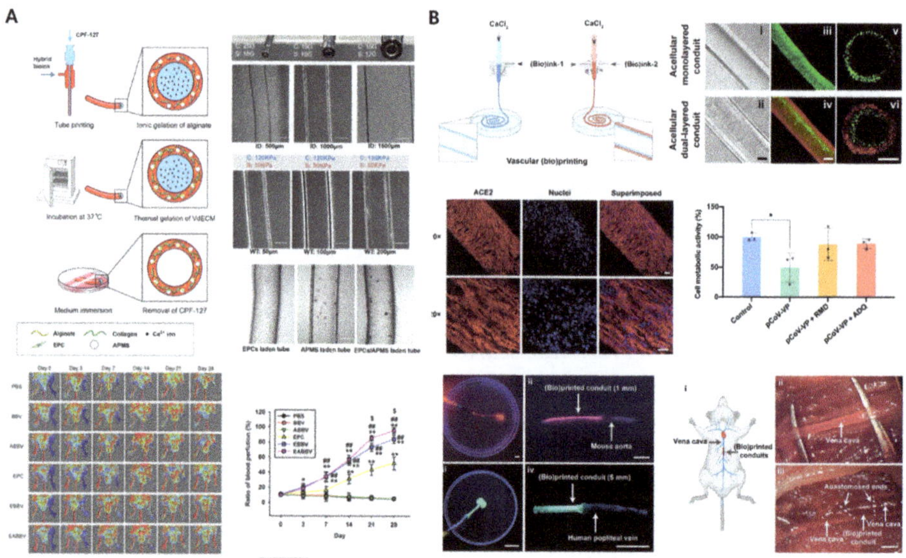

Figure 5.5. 3D coaxial bioprinting for direct fabrication of vascular graft. (A) Using coaxial cell-printing technology, vascular grafts constituted with endothelial progenitor cells and pro-angiogenic drugs were fabricated for vascular tissue regeneration. The constructed vascular graft showed therapeutic efficacy in an ischemia animal model; reproduced with permission from reference [31] John Wiley & Sons. Copyright 2017 The Authors. Published by WILEY-VCH Verlag GmbH & Co. KGaA, Weinheim. (B) Alginate-gelatin hydrogel-based vascular conduits were fabricated, which exhibited mechanically and biologically relevant features, and were implanted into vena cava to demonstrate the feasibility of the vascular graft. Reprinted with permission of AAAS from [33], copyright The Authors, some rights reserved; exclusive licensee AAAS. Distributed under a CC BY-NC 4.0 License (http://creativecommons.org/licenses/by-nc/4.0/).

developed a hybrid bioink composed of a vascular-tissue-derived ECM and alginate. The rapid cross-linking of the hydrogel responded to calcium ions from the core nozzle, and the structural stability of the tubes was maintained. Moreover, the therapeutic efficacy of the constructs against ischemic diseases was verified by blending endothelial progenitor cells with atorvastatin-loaded PLGA microspheres. Moreover, the authors applied the strategy for modeling biomimetic arterial equivalents [32]. Multilayered small-diameter vascular grafts exhibited superior patency and integration with the host abdominal aorta. Wang *et al* developed tough hydrogel-based vascular conduits using microfluidic bioprinting technology (figure 5.5(B)) [33]. The hydrogel was formulated using energy-dissipative ionically cross-linked alginate and elastic enzyme-cross-linked gelatin. The fabricated vascular conduits exhibited proper functionalities considering their mechanical properties (tensile strength, elastic modulus, and burst pressure) and endothelial barrier functions. Moreover, the feasibility of the developed vascular graft was explored through *in vivo* implantation into mouse vena cava.

Undoubtedly, tissue-engineered vascular grafts are promising regenerative medications for replacing destroyed blood vessels. With progressive technological advances, more biomimetic and functional constructs that retain appropriate biochemical and mechanical properties will be developed.

5.4 3D bioprinted superficial tissue engineering

Superficial tissues, which are located in the outermost part of the body and come in contact with foreign substances, have specific structural characteristics. For example, skin and cornea are superficial tissues. The skin has a papillary layer that regulates the body temperature via capillaries within each papilla. This functional layered skin can be reproduced using 3D bioprinting. Cubo *et al* fabricated 3D-bioprinted skin tissue equivalent consisting of dermis (plasma fibrin encapsulating human fibroblasts) and epidermis (human keratinocytes) [34]. They implanted the printed skin tissue into full-thickness circular wounds of 12 mm diameter on the dorsum of mice. The result of eight-week postgrafting showed neoangiogenesis formation similar to the capillary network found in the papillary dermis of normal skin. Kim *et al* developed a vascularized skin patch using a skin-derived dECM bioink that encapsulated endothelial progenitor cells and human adipose-derived MSCs [35]. A skin equivalent was fabricated according to the size of the cutaneous wound (diameter: 10 mm; thickness: 1 mm). They reported that this prevascularized skin patch promoted *in vivo* wound healing by accelerating wound closure, re-epithelialization, neovascularization, and blood flow. Uzel *et al* developed a multimaterial multinozzle adaptive 3D printing technology that can be used on complex substrates with varying topographies [36]. They demonstrated the potential of the direct printing on model skin wounds and structural defect repair.

The cornea has patterned lamellae in the stromal layers. The inner collagenous pattern of the corneal stroma affects its transparency. Kim *et al* fabricated transparent corneal stromal tissue using a predifferentiated keratocyte-laden cornea-derived dECM bioink and shear stress-applied extrusion-based 3D cell-printing process [37, 38]. They demonstrated the superior transparency and *in vivo* safety of cornea-derived dECM bioinks when compared to collagen used in a clinic. The printed structure replicated the native corneal macrostructure with aligned collagen fibrils, resulting in the construction of a highly mature and transparent corneal stromal equivalent. After four weeks of *in vivo* implantation, the collagen fibrils generated a lattice pattern similar to that of the human cornea, becoming more transparent. He *et al* developed an epithelium/stroma bilayer corneal implant using DLP printing technology [39]. Solutions of gelatin methacrylate and long-chain poly (ethylene glycol) diacrylate were blended with rabbit corneal epithelial cells and rabbit adipose-derived MSCs for the epithelial and stromal layers, respectively. This bilayer corneal scaffold was used in a rabbit keratoplasty model. The postoperative outcomes revealed the sealing efficacy of corneal defects, including re-epithelialization and stromal regeneration.

In summary, 3D bioprinting technology is a powerful tool for replicating the features of superficial tissues by reproducing the specific layered structures. With progressive advances, functional superficial tissues will be developed for clinical treatments.

5.5 End-of chapter problem and examples

Q1. Enumerate the different types of candidate stem cells with cardiac regenerative potential.

A. Multipotent adult stem cells and pluripotent stem cells (such as embryonic and induced pluripotent stem cells).

Q2. Describe the key features that a vascular graft must possess for successful implantation.

A. Biocompatible prostheses should retain endothelialization and possess appropriate mechanical properties, such as burst pressure, compliance, and suture retention.

Q3. Describe the advantage of 3D bioprinting for engineering superficial tissues.

A. 3D bioprinting technology can be used to replicate the specific layered structure of each superficial tissue.

References

[1] Park W, Gao G and Cho D-W 2021 Tissue-specific decellularized extracellular matrix bioinks for musculoskeletal tissue regeneration and modeling using 3D bioprinting technology *Int. J. Mol. Sci.* **22** 7837

[2] Alcala-Orozco C R, Cui X, Hooper G J, Lim K S and Woodfield T B F 2021 Converging functionality: strategies for 3D hybrid-construct biofabrication and the role of composite biomaterials for skeletal regeneration *Acta Biomater.* **132** 188–216

[3] Roddy E, DeBaun M R, Daoud-Gray A, Yang Y P and Gardner M J 2018 Treatment of critical-sized bone defects: clinical and tissue engineering perspectives *Eur. J. Orthop. Surg. Traumatol.* **28** 351–62

[4] Chae S and Cho D-W 2023 Biomaterial-based 3D bioprinting strategy for orthopedic tissue engineering *Acta Biomater.* **156** 4–20

[5] Lee J, Hong J, Kim W and Kim G H 2020 Bone-derived dECM/alginate bioink for fabricating a 3D cell-laden mesh structure for bone tissue engineering *Carbohydrate Polym.* **250** 116914
[6] Kim W and Kim G 2020 Collagen/bioceramic-based composite bioink to fabricate a porous 3D hASCs-laden structure for bone tissue regeneration *Biofabrication* **12** 015007
[7] Kang H-W, Lee S J, Ko I K, Kengla C, Yoo J J and Atala A 2016 A 3D bioprinting system to produce human-scale tissue constructs with structural integrity *Nat. Biotechnol.* **34** 312–9
[8] de Melo B A G, Jodat Y A, Mehrotra S, Calabrese M A, Kamperman T, Mandal B B, Santana M H A, Alsberg E, Leijten J and Shin S R 2019 3D printed cartilage-like tissue constructs with spatially controlled mechanical properties *Adv. Funct. Mater.* **29** 1906330
[9] Sun Y, You Y, Jiang W, Wang B, Wu Q and Dai K 2020 3D bioprinting dual-factor releasing and gradient-structured constructs ready to implant for anisotropic cartilage regeneration *Sci. Adv.* **6** eaay1422
[10] Chae S, Lee S-S, Choi Y-J, Hong D H, Gao G, Wang J H and Cho D-W 2021 3D cell-printing of biocompatible and functional meniscus constructs using meniscus-derived bioink *Biomaterials* **267** 120466
[11] Liu N *et al* 2021 Advances in 3D bioprinting technology for cardiac tissue engineering and regeneration *Bioact. Mater.* **6** 1388–401
[12] Virani S S *et al* 2021 Heart disease and stroke statistics—2021 update *Circulation* **143** e254–743
[13] Das S, Nam H and Jang J 2021 3D bioprinting of stem cell-laden cardiac patch: a promising alternative for myocardial repair *APL Bioeng.* **5** 031508
[14] Kato B, Wisser G, Agrawal D K, Wood T and Thankam F G 2021 3D bioprinting of cardiac tissue: current challenges and perspectives *J. Mater. Sci., Mater. Med.* **32** 54
[15] Wang Z, Wang L, Li T, Liu S, Guo B, Huang W and Wu Y 2021 3D bioprinting in cardiac tissue engineering *Theranostics* **11** 7948–69
[16] Jang J *et al* 2017 3D printed complex tissue construct using stem cell-laden decellularized extracellular matrix bioinks for cardiac repair *Biomaterials* **112** 264–74
[17] Park S-J *et al* 2019 Dual stem cell therapy synergistically improves cardiac function and vascular regeneration following myocardial infarction *Nat. Commun.* **10** 3123
[18] Park B-W *et al* 2020 In vivo priming of human mesenchymal stem cells with hepatocyte growth factor–engineered mesenchymal stem cells promotes therapeutic potential for cardiac repair *Sci. Adv.* **6** eaay6994
[19] Cao X, Maharjan S, Ashfaq R, Shin J and Zhang Y S 2021 Bioprinting of small-diameter blood vessels *Engineering* **7** 832–44
[20] Jones A 1997 The blood *Lancet* **349** 963
[21] Paul O, Tao J Q, Guo X and Chatterjee S 2021 The vascular system: components, signaling, and regulation *Endothelial Signaling in Vascular Dysfunction and Disease* (New York: Elsevier) pp 3–13
[22] Camasão D and Mantovani D 2021 The mechanical characterization of blood vessels and their substitutes in the continuous quest for physiological-relevant performances. A critical review *Mater. Today Bio.* **10** 100106
[23] Tucker W D, Arora Y and Mahajan K 2017 *Anatomy, Blood Vessels* (Treasure Island, FL: StatPearls Publishing)
[24] Rodrigues I C P, Kaasi A, Maciel Filho R, Jardini A L and Gabriel L P 2018 Cardiac tissue engineering: current state-of-the-art materials, cells and tissue formation *Einstein (Sao Paulo)* **16** eRB4538
[25] Fang S, Ellman D G and Andersen D C 2021 Tissue engineering of small-diameter vascular grafts and their *in vivo* evaluation in large animals and humans *Cells* **10** 713

[26] Fazal F, Raghav S, Callanan A, Koutsos V and Radacsi N 2021 Recent advancements in the bioprinting of vascular grafts *Biofabrication* **13** 032003

[27] Szklanny A A, Machour M, Redenski I, Chochola V, Goldfracht I, Kaplan B, Epshtein M, Simaan Yameen H, Merdler U and Feinberg A 2021 3D bioprinting of engineered tissue flaps with hierarchical vessel networks (VesselNet) for direct host-to-implant perfusion *Adv. Mater.* **33** 2102661

[28] Su H, Li Q, Li D, Li H, Feng Q, Cao X and Dong H 2022 A versatile strategy to construct free-standing multi-furcated vessels and a complicated vascular network in heterogeneous porous scaffolds via combination of 3D printing and stimuli-responsive hydrogels *Mater. Horizons* **9** 2393–407

[29] Norotte C, Marga F S, Niklason L E and Forgacs G 2009 Scaffold-free vascular tissue engineering using bioprinting *Biomaterials* **30** 5910–7

[30] Itoh M, Nakayama K, Noguchi R, Kamohara K, Furukawa K, Uchihashi K, Toda S, Oyama J-i, Node K and Morita S 2015 Scaffold-free tubular tissues created by a bio-3D printer undergo remodeling and endothelialization when implanted in rat aortae *PLoS One* **10** e0136681

[31] Gao G, Lee J H, Jang J, Lee D H, Kong J S, Kim B S, Choi Y J, Jang W B, Hong Y J and Kwon S M 2017 Tissue engineered bio-blood-vessels constructed using a tissue-specific bioink and 3D coaxial cell printing technique: a novel therapy for ischemic disease *Adv. Funct. Mater.* **27** 1700798

[32] Gao G, Kim H, Kim B S, Kong J S, Lee J Y, Park B W, Chae S, Kim J, Ban K and Jang J 2019 Tissue-engineering of vascular grafts containing endothelium and smooth-muscle using triple-coaxial cell printing *Appl. Phys. Rev.* **6** 041402

[33] Wang D, Maharjan S, Kuang X, Wang Z, Mille L S, Tao M, Yu P, Cao X, Lian L and Lv L 2022 Microfluidic bioprinting of tough hydrogel-based vascular conduits for functional blood vessels *Sci. Adv.* **8** eabq6900

[34] Cubo N, Garcia M, Del Canizo J F, Velasco D and Jorcano J L 2016 3D bioprinting of functional human skin: production and *in vivo* analysis *Biofabrication* **9** 015006

[35] Kim B S, Kwon Y W, Kong J-S, Park G T, Gao G, Han W, Kim M-B, Lee H, Kim J H and Cho D-W 2018 3D cell printing of *in vitro* stabilized skin model and *in vivo* pre-vascularized skin patch using tissue-specific extracellular matrix bioink: a step towards advanced skin tissue engineering *Biomaterials* **168** 38–53

[36] Uzel S G, Weeks R D, Eriksson M, Kokkinis D and Lewis J A 2022 Multimaterial multinozzle adaptive 3D printing of soft materials *Adv. Mater. Technol.* **7** 2101710

[37] Kim H, Park M-N, Kim J, Jang J, Kim H-K and Cho D-W 2019 Characterization of cornea-specific bioink: high transparency, improved *in vivo* safety *J. Tissue Eng.* **10** 2041731418823382

[38] Kim H, Jang J, Park J, Lee K-P, Lee S, Lee D-M, Kim K H, Kim H K and Cho D-W 2019 Shear-induced alignment of collagen fibrils using 3D cell printing for corneal stroma tissue engineering *Biofabrication* **11** 035017

[39] He B, Wang J, Xie M, Xu M, Zhang Y, Hao H, Xing X, Lu W, Han Q and Liu W 2022 3D printed biomimetic epithelium/stroma bilayer hydrogel implant for corneal regeneration *Bioact. Mater* **17** 234–47

IOP Publishing

Organ Printing (Second Edition)

Jinah Jang, Suhun Chae, Jungbin Yoon, Hyeonji Kim and Wonbin Park

Chapter 6

Three-dimensional bioprinting application for *in vitro* tissue/organ models

High-precision 3D bioprinting is a promising tool for developing *in vitro* models that reflect the biological and physiological functions of human tissues and organs. This chapter discusses the latest achievements in 3D bioprinting technologies for various *in vitro* tissue and organ models.

6.1 3D bioprinting of *in vitro* intestine (gut) models

The gastrointestinal tract is a continuous tubular organ responsible for transporting and digesting consumed food and absorbing nutrients and excess water. Moreover, the intestinal barriers provide physical and immunological defenses by cooperating with the intestinal tissue-specific immune system [1]. All dietary nutrients are absorbed into the blood across the highly polarized epithelial cell layer, forming the small and large intestinal mucosa. The small intestine measures approximately 6 m in length and 2.5–3.0 cm in diameter, whereas the colon measures approximately 1.5 m in length and has a 6–7.5 cm diameter [2]. Owing to the presence of villi and microvilli on the most absorptive columnar epithelial cells, the surface area of the small intestine and its absorptive capabilities are significantly enhanced. Most nutrients are transported in the small intestine, whereas the colon is primarily responsible for water and electrolyte transport. The bulk (approximately 1.5 l) of fluids and electrolytes (Na^+, Cl^-, and HCO_3^-) are transported across the small intestine to the colon; these fluids are reabsorbed in the colon, and the remaining (approximately 100 ml) leave the body through stools every day [2].

To understand the human intestinal system, physiologically relevant *in vitro* intestinal models with 3D hollow tubular structures were developed using a 3D bioprinting strategy. The *in vitro* 3D intestinal model mimics the systemic complexity of native intestinal tissue. This complex microarchitecture enables us to understand the tissue development process and intestine-related disease progression.

Han *et al* established a tissue-specific biomaterial, that is, a colon-derived dECM (colon dECM) [3]. These intestinal tissue-specific biomaterials provide encapsulated intestinal cells and organoids to maintain a significant maturation-guiding potential in human intestinal cells. Moreover, they developed a light-activated colon dECM bioink and a cell-encapsulated colon dECM bioink supplemented with ruthenium/sodium persulfate as a photoinitiator (figure 6.1(A)) [3]. The light-activated colon dECM bioink yielded improved printability; hence, it enabled the fabrication of a perfusable tubular model and achieved the simultaneous printing of multiple materials through concentrically assembled nozzles (figure 6.1(B)) [3]. Furthermore, the printed *in vitro* 3D intestinal tissue models showed spontaneous 3D morphogenesis of the human intestinal epithelium without external stimuli, which enhanced the sustainability and bio-susceptibility of the 3D printed structures for 21 days (figures 6.1(C) and (D)) [3].

Moreover, printed cells form multicellular aggregates and cysts, which subsequently differentiate into several types of enterocytes, building junctional networks [3]. This system can serve as a platform to evaluate the effects of potential drug-induced toxicity on the human intestinal tissue and to create a coculture model with commensal microbes and immune cells for future therapeutics.

The role of the human intestinal tract in host-microbe interactions has been highlighted in recent years. A trillion microorganisms comprise the human

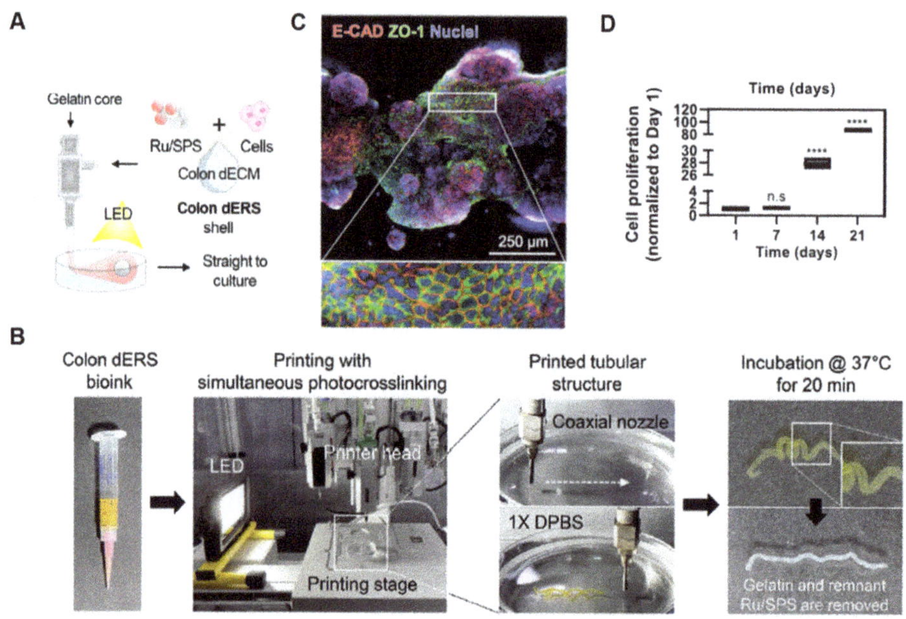

Figure 6.1. Long-term evaluation of the *in vitro* bioprinted intestine model. (A) Schematic of the 3D printing strategy. (B) Fabrication procedure of the *in vitro* bioprinted intestine model. (C) Presentative expression of junctional proteins (E-cadherin [red] and zonula occludens-1 (ZO-1) [green]) in *in vitro* bioprinted intestine model at day 21. (D) Quantitative analyses of cell proliferation of the *in vitro* model at days 1, 7, 14, and 21; reproduced with permission from reference [3] John Wiley & Sons. Copyright 2021 Wiley-VCH GmbH.

microbiome in the microenvironment of the human intestine [4]. A healthy human microbiome protects humans from diseases; however, overpopulation of pathogenic bacteria such as *Salmonella* cause diarrhea, infectious diseases, inflammatory bowel disease, and more severe colorectal cancer [5]. Cheng *et al* established an *in vitro* 3D sacrificially printed intestinal model by successfully demonstrating host cell–microbiome interactions under aerobic and anaerobic conditions [6]. They used the sacrificial printing of microchannel-embedded hydrogels to yield the designed structure and seeded an *in vitro* model with cancer coli-2 (Caco-2) cells to construct an *in vitro* 3D intestinal model (figures 6.2(A) and (B)) [6].

Furthermore, the intestinal pathogenic bacteria, *Salmonella*, was co-cultured directly with intestinal epithelial cells (host cells) in the established 3D model under aerobic and anaerobic conditions. They subsequently compared gene expression differences between aerobic and anaerobic conditions in intestinal epithelial cells and bacterial growth using dual ribonucleic acid sequencing. Consequently, inflammatory responses related to the nuclear factor kappa-light-chain enhancer of activated B cells (NF-κB) and tumor necrosis factor signaling pathways were overexpressed in the *Salmonell*a aerobic model (figure 6.2(C)) [6]. In contrast, the cell cycle-,

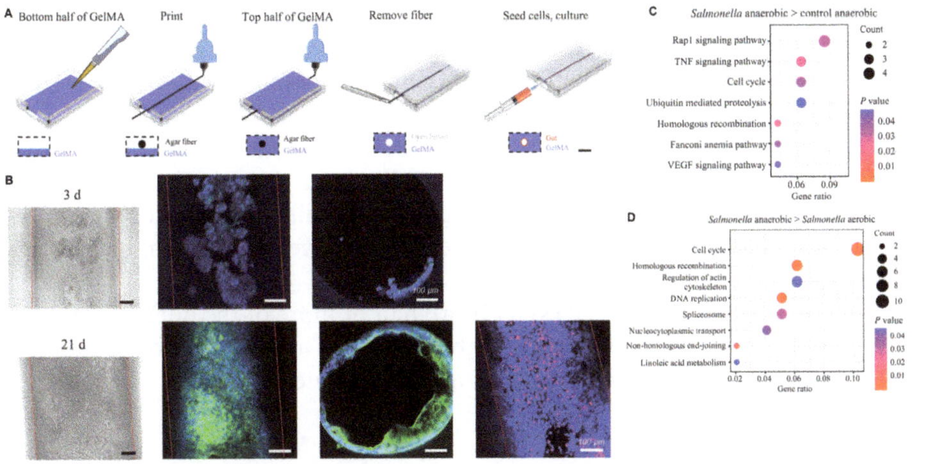

Figure 6.2. Schematic view of the typical process of sacrificial printing for fabricating a gut 3D model and evaluation of interactions between host cells and *Salmonella* in the gut 3D model. (A) Schematic view of the sacrificial printing: after semi-cross-linking using ultraviolet UV light was conducted for 10 s, a single layer of gelatin methacrylate (GelMA) solution is added to the bottom of the mold. Then, an agar fiber is printed at the predefined location; the GelMA solution is further dispersed to fill the rest of the mold and then cross-linked for 40 s. The agar fiber is finally removed from the surrounding cross-linked GelMA to allow microchannel formation. (B) Microscopic images of cancer coli-2 cells-seeded microchannels after 21 days of culture. The 3D gut model was stained with cytokeratin (green) and nuclei (blue positive Hoechst 33 342). (C) Kyoto Encyclopedia of Genes and Genomes (KEGG) and Gene Ontology (GO) pathway analyses demonstrated the enrichment of the inflammatory tumor necrosis factor signaling pathway (mediating cell survival and cell death-inducing signaling) of *Salmonella* under anaerobic conditions. (D) KEGG and GO pathway analyses demonstrated the cell cycle enrichment and deoxyribonucleic acid replication pathways in *Salmonella*-infected cells under anaerobic condition; reproduced with permission from reference [6] CC BY 4.0.

homologous recombination-, and deoxyribonucleic acid replication-related pathways were dominant in the *Salmonella* anaerobic model (figure 6.2(D)) [6]. Collectively, the *in vitro* 3D sacrificially printed intestinal model provides physiological relevance to the human intestinal environment. Such *in vitro* 3D intestinal models provide a powerful system for future in-depth gut-microbe interaction investigations.

6.2 3D bioprinting of *in vitro* kidney models

The significantly complex, bean-shaped kidney is important for eliminating body waste, removing excess drugs, balancing body fluids via solute/water reabsorption, and filtrating blood while maintaining normal blood pressure [7]. The kidney comprises three compartments: cortex, medulla, and pelvis. Each human kidney has one million nephrons in the cortex and medulla [8]. A single nephron is composed of two parts: renal corpuscle (glomerulus and Bowman's capsule) and subsequent renal tubules (proximal tubule, loop of Henle, distal tubule, and collecting ducts). Peritubular capillaries also surround the nephrons (figure 6.3) [7].

The afferent arterioles transport blood into the renal corpuscle and glomeruli. The relatively high blood pressure in the glomerular cavity causes fluids, solutes, and waste to be filtered into the Bowman's space (the interior of the Bowman's capsule). The unfiltered residual fluid is effused through the efferent arteriole and enters the peritubular capillaries and renal veins. The Bowman's capsule comprises a visceral inner layer formed by specialized cells called podocytes and an outer parietal layer composed of simple squamous epithelium. Fluids from blood in the glomerulus are ultra-filtered through several layers of the glomerular filtration membrane, resulting in the glomerular filtrate. Subsequently, the filtrate moves to the renal tubules and is further processed to form urine [9–12].

First, the proximal tubules (PTs) reabsorb half or more of the filtered sodium and glucose. Sodium reabsorption energizes the secondary active transport of numerous solutes, including glucose, amino acids, and bicarbonate. The sodium concentration

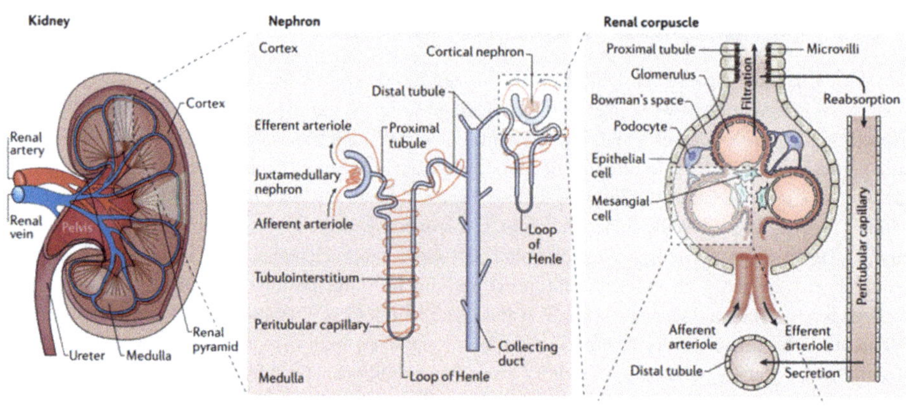

Figure 6.3. Human kidney anatomy; reproduced with permission from reference. Reproduced from [7], copyright (2018), with permission from Springer Nature.

is consistently maintained in the urinary filtrate along the PT lumen [13]. Second, in the thin limbs of the loop of Henle, the passive transportation of sodium mostly maintains the average urinary concentration, whereas the subsequent thick ascending limbs of the loop of Henle transport sodium rapidly [14]. Sodium chloride reabsorption from excess water dilutes the tubular fluid, easing the load on the urine concentrating mechanism and increasing dilution. Sodium reabsorption also provides energy for the coupled reabsorption of other cations including calcium, magnesium, potassium, and sodium [15]. Third, the distal convoluted tubules and collecting ducts play major roles in the long-term control of sodium excretion, absorption of several ions, and water reabsorption [7].

Efforts have been expended to develop *in vitro* kidney tissue models using various approaches including hollow fibers, 2D models, 3D gels, and microfluidic kidney-on-chip models. However, most previously fabricated devices have a single perfusable microchannel and contain only one type of cell. Therefore, these models cannot reflect the cellular heterogeneity of the human kidney. The 3D bioprinting method provides a new programmable route for fabricating advanced human kidney tissue models on demand.

Homan *et al* reported a 3D bioprinting method for creating convoluted 3D human renal PTs *in vitro*, which were fully embedded within an ECM and housed in perfusable tissue chips (figure 6.4(A)) [16]. These perfusable 3D human renal PTs were maintained for over two months and exhibited significantly enhanced PT epithelial cell morphology and functional properties relative to the same cells grown on 2D controls with or without perfusion (figure 6.4(B)) [16].

Furthermore, the 3D PT epithelial barrier is disrupted based on the dose of the nephrotoxin Cyclosporine A that is introduced, necessitating the development of an *in vitro* 3D renal model for drug screening and further renal disease modeling. The renal capillary network surrounds the PT of a single nephron [17]; hence, Lin *et al* created 3D vascularized PT (VasPT) models composed of adjacent conduits lined with confluent epithelium and endothelium [18]. Both 3D conduits were embedded in a permeable ECM hydrogel and independently addressed using a closed-loop perfusion system to investigate the fundamental renal reabsorption similar to that in native kidney tissue [18]. In particular, the active tubular-adjacent vascular exchange of solutes was recapitulated in a 3D VasPT model. Using this *in vitro* 3D VasPT model, the key functions of the PT (glucose reabsorption and renal epithelium–endothelium crosstalk) were confirmed as a function of time. Under hyperglycemic conditions, mature 3D PTs demonstrated enhanced glucose reabsorption on day 13 [18]. Moreover, Cy5-labeled human serum albumin was also successfully moved across the 3D PT model to the adjacent *in vitro* 3D vasculature [18].

Furthermore, using a kidney-specific bioink (porcine kidney-derived dECM mixed with viable renal-specific cells) and coaxial cell-printing techniques, multiple 3D renal-associated models were developed in the form of PT-on-a-chip and glomerulus-on-a-chip. Singh *et al* used a coaxial 3D cell-printing technique and presented microfluidic hollow tubes to recapitulate the tubular-vascular renal parenchyma composed of renal tubular epithelial and endothelial cells. Moreover, they developed a functional hybrid bioink (3K1A hybrid bioink by blending a

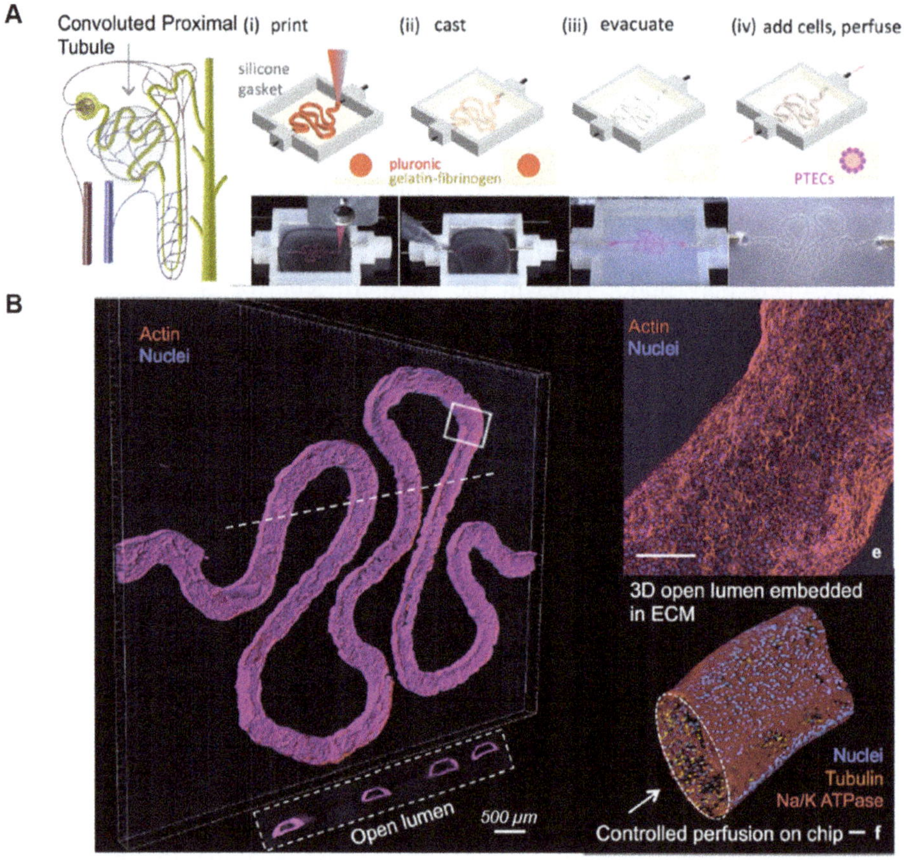

Figure 6.4. *In vitro* 3D convoluted renal proximal tubule on the chip. (A) Schematic for fabricating 3D convoluted, perfusable proximal tubules in a nephron. The fugitive ink is first printed on a gelatin-fibrinogen extracellular matrix (ECM); then, the fugitive ink is evacuated to create an open tubule after casting the complete mold. Next, proximal tubular epithelial cells (PTECs) are seeded within the hollow tubule and perfused. (B) Magnified view of PTEC channel. The transport methodology in the proximal tubule (Na/K ATPase) is stained in red. Primary cilia of PTECs are shown as orange-colored acetylated tubulin; reproduced with permission from reference [16] CC BY 4.0.

3% [w/v] kidney-derived dECM solution with 1% [w/v] alginate). Moreover, other renal proximal tubular epithelial cells (RPTECs) and human umbilical vein endothelial cells (HUVECs) were added to the hybrid bioink for the subsequent printing of 3D PTs and vessels, respectively (figures 6.5(A) and (B)) [19]. The hybrid bioink inherits the microenvironments of vascularized native kidney tissue and yields immediate cross-linkable characteristics to optimize cellular function and enhance long-term hollow tubular structural integrity. After 14 days of flow perfusion, RPTECs and HUVECs encapsulated in 3D bioprinted tubules were fully matured by increasing the expression of an epithelial glucose transporter (sodium-glucose cotransporter-2) in 3D RPTEC tubes and endothelial junction proteins (CD31) in 3D HUVEC tubes (figures 6.5(C) and (D)) [19]. After measuring the penetrating

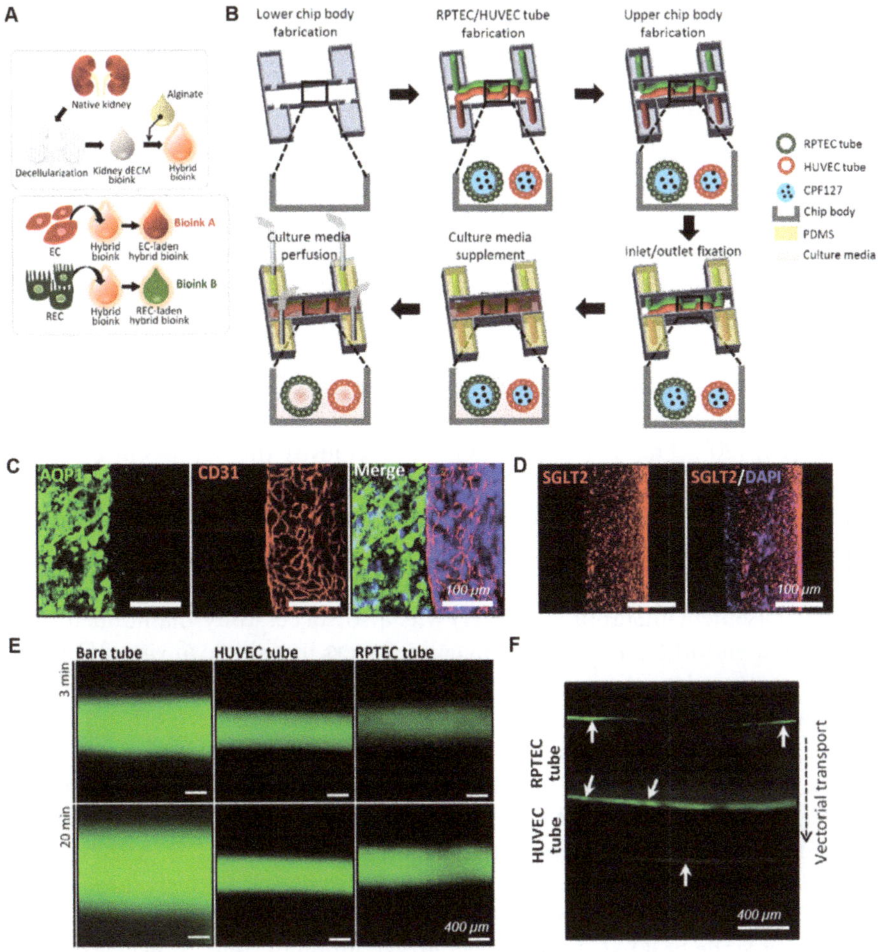

Figure 6.5. Schematic of research and functional validation of kidney-specific dECM (KdECM) bioink and KdECM bioink-based printing of 3D vascularized renal proximal tubule-on-a-chip. (A) Schematic of KdECM bioink. Decellularization of KdECM hydrogel, and further renal epithelial cells and endothelial cells were encapsulated into KdECM hydrogel to form bioinks. (B) Schematic illustration of the fabrication steps of vascularized renal proximal tubule-on-a-chip. The coaxial printed proximal tubule (renal PTEC (RPTEC) tube) and vessel (human umbilical vein endothelial cell (HUVEC) tube) were located in a 3D printed model, and further perfusion was performed on the 3D model. (C) and (D) Expression of vessel-specific CD31, proximal-tubule-specific Aquaporin-1, and SGLT2 was present on the vascularized renal proximal tubule-on-a-chip for 28 days. (E) Perfusion of 70 kDa fluorescein isothiocyanate (FITC)-conjugated dextran demonstrates reduced permeabilities of barriers in RPTEC and HUVEC tubes when compared to those of the bare tube. (F) After perfusion of FITC-albumin through the RPTEC tube for 1 h, albumin (green) was accumulated in the adjacent HUVEC tube; reproduced with permission from reference [19], copyright (2020), with permission from Elsevier.

ability of fluorescein isothiocyanate (FITC)-conjugated 70 kDa dextran across the epithelium to the endothelium, they confirmed the successful enhancement of the integrity of the proximal tubular epithelial and vascular endothelial barriers on a 3D vascularized renal PT-on-a-chip (figures 6.5(E) and (F)) [19].

Moreover, the novel bioink and 3D coaxial cell-printing technique can provide extra complexity, ranging from printing monolayered tubular structures to bilayered renal tubular 3D structures. Recently, Singh *et al* established a bilayered human glomerular microvessel-on-a-chip (bGOAC) (figure 6.6(A)) [20]. This *in vitro* 3D human glomerular model was fabricated using a customized hybrid bioink (3% [w/v] kidney-specific dECM mixed with 1% [w/v] sodium alginate) and coaxial cell-printing technology. Thus, the fabricated functional bGOAC recapitulated the bilayers arranged explicitly with the glomerular endothelium (inner layer containing glomerular endothelial cells [GEs]) and podocyte-lined layers (outer layer) (figure 6.6(B)) [20]. This perfusable bGOAC achieves the successful coculture of primary human podocytes and GEs; after seven days of flow perfusion, the expressions of vascular endothelial-specific marker CD31, podocyte-specific marker nephrin, and the tight junction zonula occludens-1 were enhanced within layers of the coaxial cell-printed bGOAC (figure 6.6(C)) [20]. Furthermore, the intervening glomerular basement membrane (GBM) was also successfully maintained between the glomerular endothelium and podocyte line layers in a single *in vitro* 3D bGOAC. Abundant major protein components of the GBM (human collagen type IV and laminin) were also observed on a perfusable bGOAC (figure 6.6(D)) [20]. These three key features enable bGOAC to perform *in vivo* human glomerulus-like functions, such as glomerular filtration and cellular crosstalk between GEs, the intervening GBM, and the highly specialized podocytes. Furthermore, a characteristic function of the *in vivo* glomerular filtration barrier, that is, selective permeability, was obtained using an *in vitro* 3D bGOAC model. Relatively large molecules (albumin and dextran) were predominantly retained (approximately 99% in the perfusate) inside the bGOAC tubule. In contrast, inulin (a small molecule) was freely diffused across the GBM from the inner bGOAC to the outer urinary component (figure 6.6(E)) [20].

Multiple fabrication strategies of single *in vitro* organ models can be combined by utilizing advanced 3D bioprinting techniques to develop an integrative *in vitro* multiorgan model. The 3D printing techniques and microfluidics can be used to structurally and functionally connect two independent organ modules. Consequently, the enhanced connectivity with organs enables the recapitulation of substance metabolic movement, biological and physiological cross-communication among organs, and multiorgan-related disease modeling. Recently, the development of a functional multiorgan-on-a-chip based on advanced engineering technologies has been actively studied to understand the physiological mechanisms of organ–organ communication and integrative disease diagnosis (a complex disease diagnosed in two organs). Secondary hyperoxaluria (SH) is a multifactorial disorder that results in kidney stone disease due to an abnormally high concentration of oxalates absorbed from the inflamed intestinal epithelium [21–23]. Yoon *et al* developed an *in vitro* multiorgan model exhibiting the enhanced functional interconnection

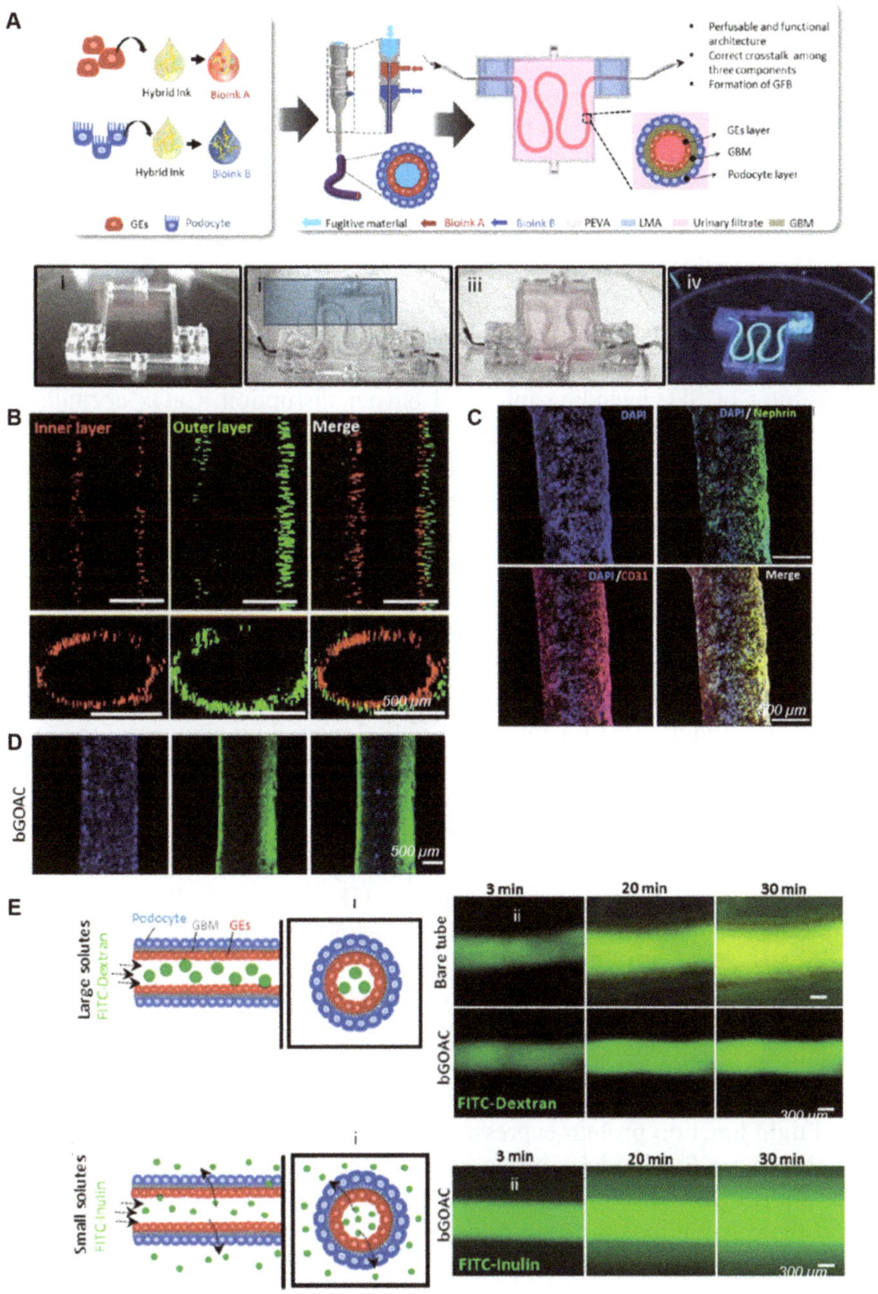

Figure 6.6. Illustration of the glomerular research strategy and functional assessment of the *in vitro* 3D bilayered human glomerular microvessel-on-a-chip (bGOAC). (A) Kidney tissue-specific hybrid bioink formation including glomerular endothelial cells and podocytes. Schematic representation of the bGOAC fabrication steps, including (i) 3D printed poly(ethylene-vinyl acetate)-based chip body, (ii, iii, iv) coaxial cell-printed bilayer glomerular microvessel connected by the microfluidic system. (B) Representative cross-sectional confocal image views of the bilayered glomerular microvessel (inner [red] and outer [green] layers).

(C) Matured bilayers expressed by enhanced vascular endothelial-specific marker CD31 (red) and podocyte-specific marker nephrin (green). (D) Tight junction (ZO-1; green) signals were thoroughly expressed along the matured bilayers of bGOAC. (E) Large FITC-conjugated dextran shows reduced diffusion of large solutes from the bGOAC and significantly decreased diffusion permeability when compared to the bare tube (upper). Small-sized inulin-FITC-enhanced diffusibility of the bilayer glomerular microvessel to the surrounding microenvironment (lower); reproduced with permission from reference [20].

between the intestinal epithelium and a vascularized renal PT by printing two compartmentalized organs together (figure 6.7(A)) [24]. The *in vitro* multiorgan model highlights the dynamic pathophysiological interactions between the native intestine and kidney and provides a tool for recapitulating the critical pathophysiological features of SH, including intestinal barrier disruption, CaOx crystallization, and crystal-induced PT injuries (figure 6.7(B)) [24]. The tubular-shaped *in vitro* vascularized proximal model was printed with kidney-derived dECM bioink mixed with human proximal tubular epithelial cells (HK-2; for *in vitro* 3D PT) and GEs (for adjacent *in vitro* 3D peritubular renal vessels). This vascularized PT module resembles a native nephron-like structure: a PT surrounded by capillary networks [17].

Furthermore, human intestinal epithelial cells (Caco-2 cells) were seeded on the intestinal barrier in a transwell interconnected to the PT module. On day 7, the fully matured *in vitro* intestinal and renal epithelium modules were further disrupted by a perfusion inflammation inducer, TNF-α, to demonstrate the pathophysiological features of SH (figures 6.7(C) and (D)) [24]. Upon fluid flow into the *in vitro* multiorgan model, the oxalate in the perfusate moved sequentially from the permeable intestinal epithelium (*in vitro* intestinal module) to the lumen of the 3D PT and successfully formed fluid-flow-behavior-dependent CaOx crystals (figure 6.7(E)) [24]. The formed renal crystals induced the damage of a vascularized PT module, exhibiting the increased death of HK-2-lined 3D PT epithelium and releasing the pro-inflammatory cytokines such as *NF-κB*, *Interleukin (IL)-6*, *IL-1β*, *TNF-α*, and *IL-8* (figures 6.7(F) and (G)) [24].

Furthermore, the efficacy of the *in vitro* 3D SH disease model as a drug-testing platform was validated by assessing the CaOx crystal dissolution by perfusing the device with trisodium citrate (TC) and grape seed extract (GSE). After drug treatment, the disturbed intestinal and proximal tubular epithelia are recovered by increased tight junction protein expression [24]. Most significantly, the microfluidics applied to *in vitro* SH model actively allowed the drug and CaOx precipitates to interface thoroughly. Therefore, CaOx crystals began to dissolve when TC was bound to the calcium ions at the surface of the CaOx crystals [24]. The therapeutic effect of GSE on the CaOx kidney stone disease was validated by observing reduced inflammation (decreased expression of pro-inflammatory cytokines IL-6, IL-8, and TNF-α) and enhanced antioxidant activities (increased expression of antioxidant transcripts glutathione-disulfide reductase, superoxide dismutase 1, superoxide dismutase 2, and glutathione peroxidase 2) [24]. In conclusion, this functionally optimized *in vitro* multiorgan model can be actively utilized as a promising platform for discovering integrative therapeutics in a single assay.

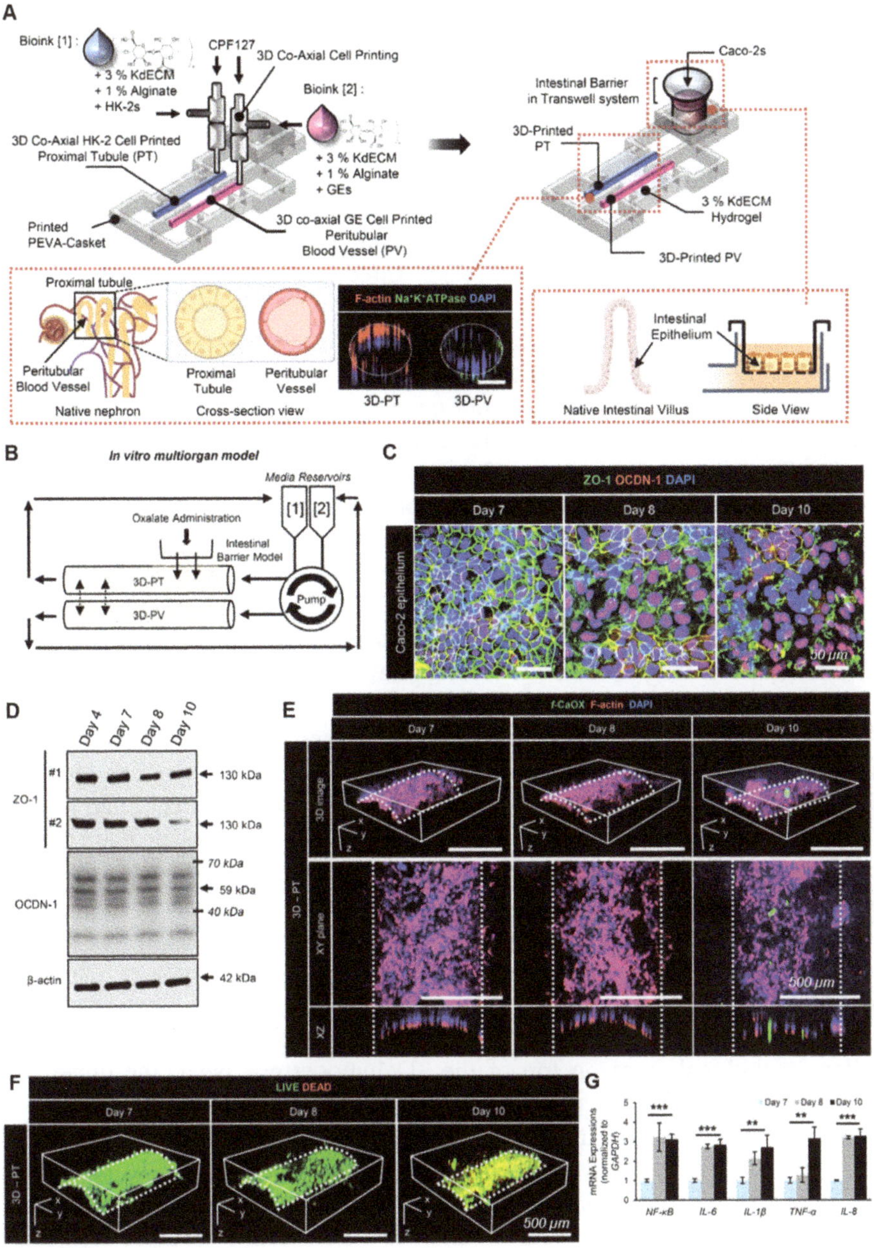

Figure 6.7. Bioengineering of integrative *in vitro* multiorgan model. (A) Schematic progress for biofabricating intestinal barrier and vascularized PT integrated humans in the *in vitro* multiorgan model. (B) Description of perfusate flows inside *in vitro* multiorgan model. (C) Images of calcium oxalate crystal-induced intestinal damage. (D) Immunoblot analyses of Caco-2 epithelium integrities of *in vitro* multiorgan model. (E) Images of calcium oxalate crystal-induced proximal tubule epithelium damages. (F) Live/dead assay analyses of proximal tubule epithelium after inducing calcium oxalate crystal precipitation. (G) Gene expressions of inflammatory cytokines-related genes in proximal tubule module of *in vitro* multiorgan model. Reproduced from reference [24], with the permission of AIP Publishing.

6.3 3D bioprinting of *in vitro* skin and adipose tissue models

The largest organ in our body (accounting for approximately 15% of the total adult body weight), that is, the human skin, accounts for approximately 15% of the entire adult body weight and has an average thickness of 2.5 mm [25]. The skin provides a primary barrier function and protects the skin against external radiation, chemicals, UV light, mechanical damage, and microorganisms. The surface of the skin also prevents excess water loss from our body to maintain our body temperature in a normal range [25]. The skin comprises three layers: epidermis, dermis, and subcutaneous tissue [26]. Densely packed keratinocytes characterize the upper stratified epidermal region, which achieves the barrier function of the skin [27]. Collagen fibers with low concentrations of fibroblasts are present in the lower dermal area, and the upper papillary dermal area is characterized by densely packed types III and I collagen fibers [28]. The dermal fibroblasts release key ECM proteins (type I collagen, type IV collagen, laminin, fibronectin, and elastin) and growth factors that promote cell-to-ECM interactions and cell-to-cell communication [28]. The dermis lies on the subcutaneous tissue or panniculus and contains small lobes of fat cells known as lipocytes. Such animal models can provide an effective testing platform owing to the similarity of their skin with human skin; however, discrepancies in genetics and controversial ethical issues still exist [29–31]. Therefore, an *in vitro* alternative drug or cosmetic testing platform that recapitulates the structural complexity of the human skin is required.

Although previous skin-cell-printed patches have shown potential in the fabrication of functional skin equivalents, multiple 3D printing technologies can increase the complexity of the skin anatomy (containing all three compartments of native skin: the epidermis, dermis, and hypodermis) inside an *in vitro* 3D skin model. The 3D printing technologies enable conventional construction by precisely localizing multiple types of cells and biomaterials [32]. Adding a perfusable vascular channel to trilayered skin equivalents promotes *in vitro* skin tissue maturation. According to the fabrication strategies of Kim *et al*, a pre-adipocyte-embedded adipose–fibrinogen hybrid bioink was initially printed to form a hypodermal compartment [33]. Moreover, a vascular bioink composed of HUVECs and thrombin in a 10% gelatin hydrogel was printed in a hollow, cylindrical form on top of the 3D hypodermis. Next, the upper dermal compartment was added by extruding the human dermis fibroblast-encapsulated skin fibrinogen hybrid bioink. Finally, the primary human epidermal keratocytes were distributed over the top using an inkjet module for 3D bioprinting (figure 6.8(A)) [33]. When compared to native human skin, the fabricated *in vitro* 3D skin model avoided dramatic structural shrinkage and maintained three distinct compartments during long-term culture (figure 6.8(B)) [33]. Kim *et al* also confirmed that *in vitro* 3D skin models closely reflect native human skin by demonstrating a comparable expression of the tumor protein p63 in the 3D epidermis and keratin 19 (K19) in the 3D hypodermis (figure 6.8(B)) [33]. The *in vivo* p63 plays an essential role in initiating epithelial stratification and maintaining the proliferative potential of basal keratinocytes in the matured epidermis [34]. Simultaneously, K19 indicates mature adipocytes in native human hypodermis [35]. Therefore, this advanced *in vitro* 3D skin model can be a

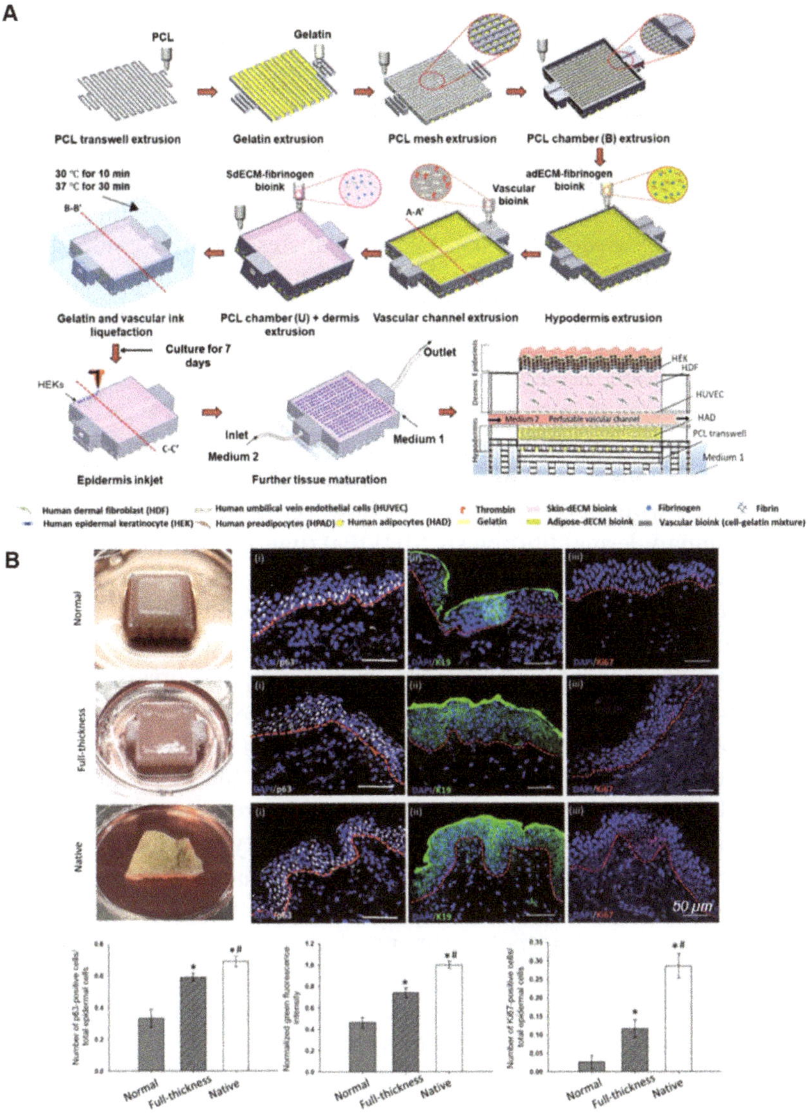

Figure 6.8. 3D cell-printing process for *in vitro* 3D full-thickness skin model fabrication. A. Schematic diagram exhibiting step-by-step fabrication process of *in vitro* 3D full-thickness skin model. The *in vitro* 3D full-thickness skin model comprises printed hypodermis, dermis, and epidermis, including 3D vasculature. B. When compared to the native skin tissue, the *in vitro* 3D full-thickness skin model also successfully recapitulated the hypodermis, dermis, and epidermis dermis. All groups were stained with p63 (white), keratin 19 (green), and Ki67 (red), and each fluorescence intensity is thoroughly quantified using graphs; reproduced with permission from reference [33] John Wiley & Sons. Copyright 2018 WILEY-VCH Verlag GmbH & Co. KGaA, Weinheim.

reliable platform for further investigation of the mechanisms in pathological research and skin-related disease modeling.

Based on the 3D cell-printing technique, Kim *et al* further modeled an *in vitro* 3D diseased skin tissue by recapitulating the pathophysiological characteristics of type 2 diabetes: increased insulin resistance, vascular dysfunction, adipose hypertrophy, and released pro-inflammatory responses [36]. Patients with type 2 diabetes have increased insulin resistance, which can lead to poor blood circulation and hyperglycemia (high blood glucose levels). Type 2 diabetes can also cause serious skin health problems with diabetic dermopathy, diabetic blister, diabetic rash, fungal infections, delayed wound healing, and skin itching [37, 38]. Therefore, diabetic patients with damaged skin can easily develop an ulcer at a high risk of infection, and despite this pathological seriousness, an effective cure for type 2 diabetes-related skin problems has not yet been established [39]. A 3D *in vitro* type 2 diabetic skin model was developed according to a previously described biofabrication method (figure 6.9(A)) [36]. This *in vitro* 3D diseased skin platform was primarily composed of three skin layers with blood vessels (BVs); however, the dermal layer was replaced with diabetic human dermal fibroblasts (dHDFs) (figure 6.9(B)) [36]. An additional wound was physically created via needle insertion during epidermal maturation.

The glucose uptake after insulin perfusion decreased in the *in vitro* 3D type 2 diabetic skin model; hence, the diabetes-induced dermis successfully demonstrated insulin resistance *in vitro* [36]. Furthermore, the size of lipid droplets of adipocytes in the hypodermis was also elevated by increasing the excess glucose storage, which led the *in vitro* 3D model to have a status of adipose hypertrophy (figure 6.9(C)) [36]. Finally, the elevated releases of IL-6 and TNF-α from the perfusate in the hyperglycemic condition confirmed that the inflammatory response, a diabetic pathophysiology, can be mimicked within an *in vitro* 3D type 2 diabetic skin model (figure 6.9(D)) [36]. Moreover, the diabetes-induced inflammatory responses in the perfusate were alleviated after perfusing an *in vitro* 3D type 2 diabetic skin model with the first-line agents for the treatment of diabetes, such as metformin and eicosapentaenoic acid (figure 6.9(E)) [29, 36, 40]. Therefore, this *in vitro* 3D-engineered diabetic skin model can be used as an advanced drug-testing platform to validate the efficacy of potential diabetes treatments.

In humans, adipose tissues are observed in various locations, such as beneath the skin, around the brain- and liver-like internal organs, bone marrow, intermuscular system, and breasts [41]. Adipose deposition is primarily responsible for energy homeostasis and promotes metabolic communication between internal organs in humans [42]. The adipose tissue also protects the body from harmful external cues and is insulated against dramatic temperature changes. The importance of understanding the role of adipose tissue has gradually increased because hormones or cytokines released from mature adipocytes are involved in the systemic performance of major organs [43–46]. Using environmentally controlled in-bath 3D bioprinting, Ahn *et al* established a densely packed adipose tissue (DPAT) construct [47]. A pre-adipocyte-laden 1.5% adipose-derived dECM (AdECM) bioink was extruded in an environmentally controlled bath suspension composed of a hybrid bioink (1% alginate and 1.5% AdECM mixed bioink) (figure 6.10(A)) [47]. This 3D

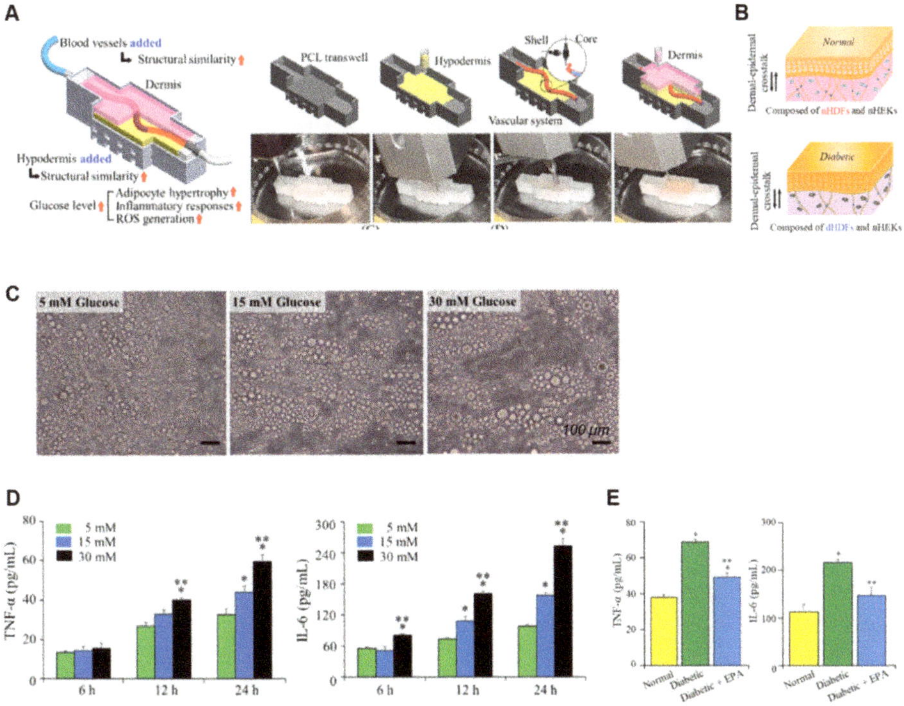

Figure 6.9. Engineering normal and diabetic skin models using a polycaprolactone (PCL) transwell system and devised wounded skin model through 3D cell-printing process. (A) Fabrication of engineering diabetic skin model via using a PCL transwell system and 3D cell printing. Additional perfusable vessels were embedded in the hypodermal compartment. (B) Schematic illustrations that show cellular compositions in normal/diabetic skin models. In *in vitro* 3D diseased skin platform, the dermal compartment was placed with diabetic human dermal fibroblast. (C) Micrographs of differentiated-diabetic preadipocytes cultured with different glucose levels. Pre-adipocyte sizes increased as the concentrations of treated glucose were increased. (D) Measurement of the pro-inflammatory cytokines (TNF-α and Interleukin-6 [IL-6]) from the perfusate samples containing different glucose levels. (E) After treatment using eicosapentaenoic acid (anticancer drug) in the *in vitro* 3D model, the inflammatory responses were reduced when accessing the release of pro-inflammatory cytokines (TNF-α and IL-6); reproduced with permission from reference [36], copyright (2021), with permission from Elsevier.

bioprinting method enabled the dense packing of printed preadipocytes in a limited area without cell migration. It also promoted pre-adipocyte maturation to mature adipocytes by significantly increasing the secretion of representative adipokines such as adiponectin and leptin (figures 6.10(B) and (C)) [47]. Moreover, the successful recapitulation of obesity-induced inflamed adipose tissue *in vitro* was established by coculturing obese DPAT constructs with monocytes (figure 6.10(D)) [47]. Moreover, a CD-68-positive M1 macrophage surrounds mature adipocytes in a crown-like structure, an outstanding feature of the early stage of chronic low-grade inflammation in adipose tissue *in vivo* (figure 6.10(E)) [47–49]. In conclusion, the functional, 3D bioprinted normal and obese DPAT constructs have the potential to replace animal-based studies and search for promising therapeutics to overcome obesity-related diseases.

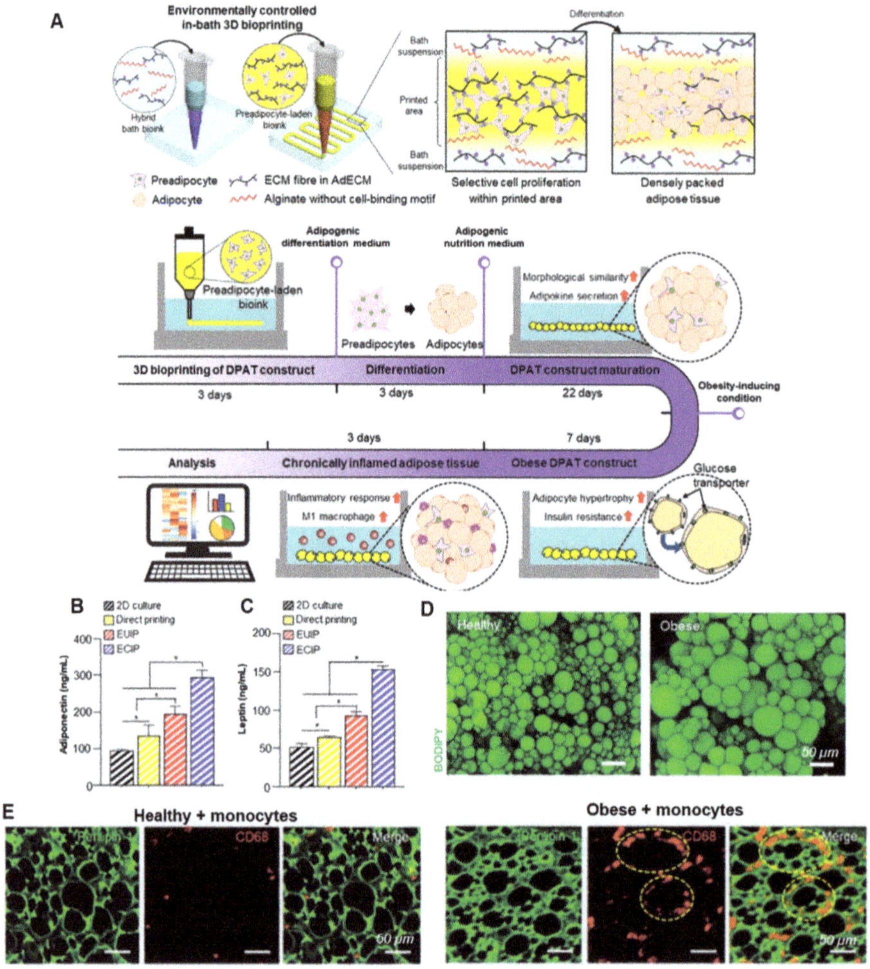

Figure 6.10. Conceptual design for environmentally controlled in-bath 3D bioprinting (ECIP) for constructing the densely packed adipose tissue (DPAT) model and analyzing adipose tissue-equivalents created by conventional 3D in-bath adipose tissue engineering. (A) Schematic illustration of the workflow for biofabricating 3D DPAT construct using the method of ECIP. (B) and (C) When compared to 2D culture, directing printing, and environmentally uncontrolled in-bath 3D bioprinting groups, the releases of adiponectin and leptin were enhanced on the matured adipocytes in the ECIP groups. (D) When compared to the adipose tissue in healthy conditions, the size of adipose tissue in the obesity-induced DPAT construct was enlarged. Moreover, the green-colored boron-dipyrromethene revealed mature adipocytes. (E) Recapitulation of chronic low-grade adipose inflammation within an *in vitro* 3D DPAT construct via monocyte coculture. Under the obese condition (Obese + monocyte group), monocytes (CD68-positive inflammatory cells; red) were recruited around matured adipocytes via crown-like morphologies (indicated using yellow-dashed circles); reproduced with permission from reference [47] John Wiley & Sons. Copyright 2022 Wiley-VCH GmbH.

6.4 Three-dimensional bioprinting of *in vitro* blood vessel models

BVs have significantly complex structures that depend on their location and function, as mentioned in section 5.3.1. The BVs extending throughout the body circulate key substances to mediate biological, chemical, and biophysical interactions between various cells and maintain homeostasis in the body [50]. However, our understanding of the physiological features or pathological progression of vascular tissues is at an infant stage, although prerequisites for establishing effective methods for disease treatment and prevention involve identifying the pathophysiological phenomena [51]. Conventionally, animal models have been used to predict clinical outcomes by elucidating the underlying molecular mechanisms and testing therapeutic strategies. However, in addition to species differences and ethical issues, the need for human-specific *in vitro* models has increased drastically. Therefore, various interdisciplinary strategies have been suggested to provide insights into the modeling of healthy and diseased human tissues and organs and finding candidate drugs for clinical trials.

In this chapter, 3D printed *in vitro* BV models are discussed. For the successful modeling of vascular tissues *in vitro*, several key factors, including cellular, biochemical, structural, and mechanical cues, should be considered. In particular, interactions between endothelial cells and the surrounding biophysical microenvironment should be investigated to engineer models, because the main performance of BVs is the based on the endothelial function [52, 53]. Therefore, most research has focused on vasculogenesis, endothelial barrier properties, angiogenesis, transendothelial transport and migration, and cell–cell or cell–ECM interactions. The endothelial cells regulate molecular transport and cellular migration. In response to external stimuli, such as inflammation or hypoxia, endothelial cells support immune cell trafficking and form new BVs through angiogenesis [54]. Conversely, cellular interactions resulting from cellular organization, such as coculture or the alignment of multiple cell types, can alter vessel stability and junctional barrier tightness. Cytokines, such as TNF-α, or growth factors, such as vascular endothelial and basic fibroblast growth factors, which are secreted from the surrounding cells can induce vascular permeability changes. Moreover, structural and biophysical factors, including ECM alignment, stiffness, and hemodynamic flow, can remodel cellular morphology.

To elucidate the performance of BVs *in vitro* using 3D bioprinting, multiple factors should be considered, such as biomaterials, including multiple cell types and biocompatible bioinks, and the dimensional design of the vascular architecture, cellular alignment, and molecular gradient. Typically, *in vitro* vascular tissue models are fabricated by indirect or direct bioprinting. Sacrificial bioprinting, a classical indirect method, involves the fabrication of tubular constructs using fugitive biomaterials, such as Pluronic F127, carbohydrate glass, gelatin, and alginate [40, 55, 56]. Through the dissolution or physical aspiration of fugitive biomaterials, unnecessary parts are eliminated, leaving perfusable channels. ECs were seeded into interconnected hollow channels to generate the endothelial layer. Kolesky *et al* developed thick vascularized tissues (>1 cm) by drawing a fugitive ink composed of Pluronic F127 and thrombin in a hydrogel bath consisting of fibrinogen, gelatin, and

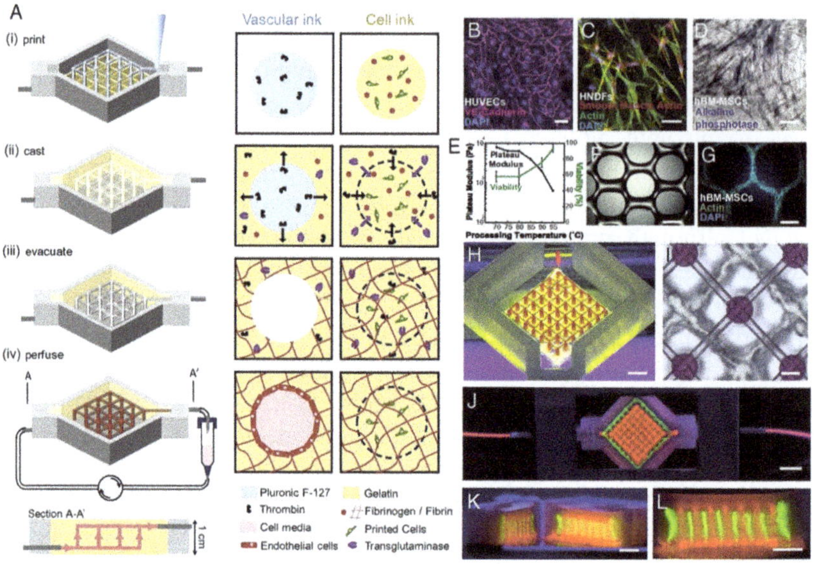

Figure 6.11. Three-dimensional bioprinting of a complex vascular network using Pluronic F127. Fugitive vascular ink created using Pluronic F127 and thrombin and cell-laden ink containing gelatin, fibrinogen, and cells were printed to fabricate complex vascular network. In the constructs, endothelial cells, fibroblasts, mesenchymal stem cells matured [40]; reproduced with permission of National Academy of Sciences.

calcium chloride (figure 6.11) [40]. Upon printing, cross-linking was achieved by diffused enzymes, and the removal of the fugitive material resulted in complex vascular channels. These tubes promote the differentiation of hMSCs toward an osteogenic lineage by delivering the necessary growth factors.

Song *et al* patterned complex microchannels with adamantane-blended hyaluronic acid in beta-cyclodextrin-blended hyaluronic acid bath [57]. Straight, stenotic, and spiral microchannels could be produced with high fidelity. For an angiogenic sprouting assay, channels were fabricated in parallel, and angiogenic growth factors were perfused to form the concentration gradient. Following the direction of the gradient, endothelial cells invaded the hydrogel and angiogenic sprouting was observed. Although the vascular functionality could be successfully investigated, the fabrication process was complicated, and a simpler strategy is required.

The complex structure of the vascular tissue can be recapitulated using a direct printing strategy. Grigoryan *et al* developed multivascular networks within biocompatible hydrogels using ethylene glycol diacrylate, which is a photopolymerizable hydrogel [58]. The authors investigated the efficacy of intervascular interstitial transport by perfusing human red blood cells into a 3D vascular topology and observed oxygen delivery phenomena. Conversely, the dimensional controllability of 3D bioprinting technology allows the investigation of the continuity between the shape of the BV and pathological development resulting from flow divergence. Gao *et al* developed perfusable BVs using coaxial bioprinting technology and investigated the inflammatory responses of the endothelium to external stimuli [59]. By applying this technology, the authors also fabricated multilayered artery equivalents via in-bath coaxial cell-printing technology for investigating the geometrical effects of BVs on development of atherosclerosis (figure 6.12) [60]. Based on the coculture condition and local turbulent flow condition, the pathological initiation was promoted. Moreover, the dose-dependent therapeutic effects of atorvastatin, a cholesterol-lowering drug, were demonstrated in this model. Previous studies have demonstrated the potential of modeling the physiological and pathological features of BVs *in vitro*.

BVs are also involved in the development of various other diseases, such as tumor metastasis. A tumor is an abnormal cell mass with dozens of malignant mutations. Genetic alterations are related to its pathological features including uncontrollable proliferation, metabolism, metastasis, and chemoresistance. The heterogeneous cellular compositions generate a tumor-favorable microenvironment, including cellular (tumor-associated fibroblasts, endothelial cells, and immune cells), biochemical (ECM components, cytokines, and chemoattractants), and mechanical

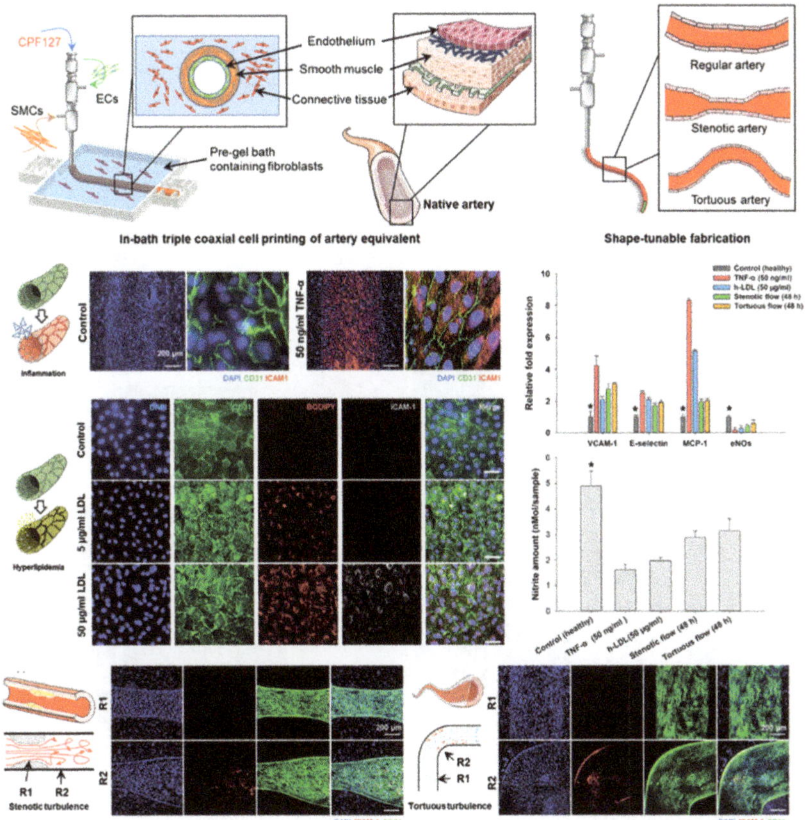

Figure 6.12. Three-dimensional bioprinting for direct fabrication of *in vitro* vascular tissue models. (A) Using in-bath triple coaxial bioprinting technology, a triple-layered BV could be fabricated. Controlling the printing parameters achieved the generation of stenotic BV for the investigation of atherosclerosis initiation. Moreover, effective drug candidates could be tested using the model. [60]; reproduced with permission of John Wiley & Sons. Copyright 2020 Wiley-VCH GmbH.

(solid stress, fluid stress, and stiffness) cues. Kim *et al* verified the applicability of an in-bath printing strategy for the one-step fabrication of metastatic cancer models possessing vasculatures and tumor spheroids (figure 6.13(A)) [61]. Metastasis-associated changes in adjacent and distal regions can be studied by controlling the distance between BVs and malignant cells. The ability of 3D bioprinting technology to recapitulate the native microenvironment can be utilized to study cancer pathogenesis and metastasis. Moreover, Cho *et al* fabricated a blood-lymphatic integrated system with heterogeneous melanoma spheroids to investigate the effects of combined targeted therapies (figure 6.13(B)) [62]. The hallmark events of melanoma metastasis, including stromal interaction, invasion, and intravasation through the constructed vascular structure were recapitulated in the model. Yi *et al* developed a human glioblastoma-on-a-chip for the identification of precision cancer medicine for patient-specific treatments (Figure 6.13(C)) [63, 64]. The generation of tubule networks through angiogenesis was observed by printing endothelial cells surrounding the hypoxic glioblastoma constructs. Using patient-derived glioblastoma cells, patient-specific resistance to treatment with concurrent chemoradiation and temozolomide treatment was evaluated, demonstrating that the best drug combination

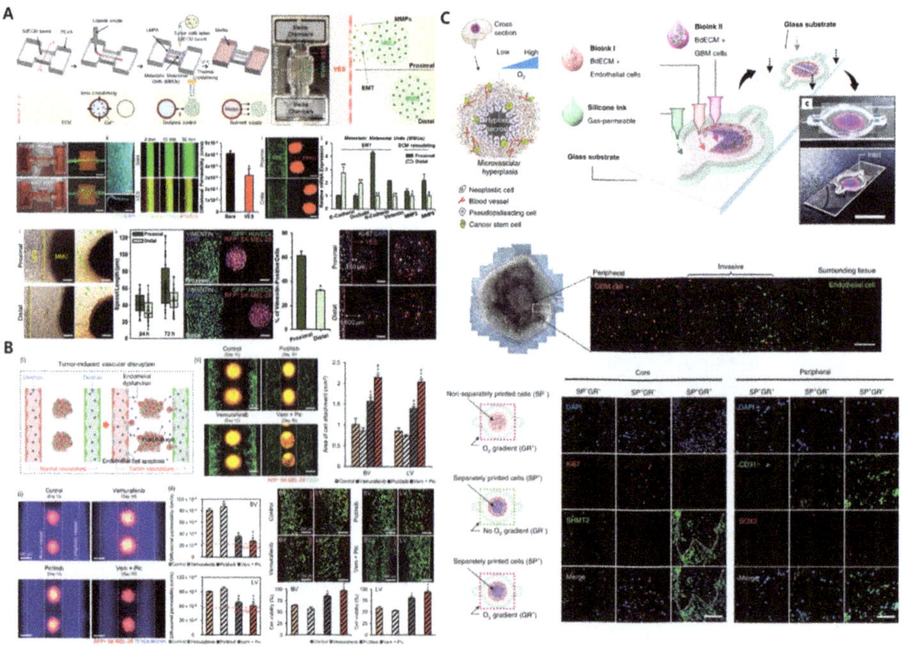

Figure 6.13. 3D bioprinting of *in vitro* vascularized cancer models. (A) Using in-bath coaxial bioprinting technology, a BV with fully mature endothelium was constructed to investigate the interaction between the BV and cancer spheroids; reproduced with permission from reference [61] John Wiley & Sons. Copyright 2021 Wiley-VCH GmbH. (B) As an advanced approach, a BV and LV pair was fabricated to demonstrate the metastatic progression in drug resistance of melanoma; reproduced with permission from reference [62] CC BY 4.0. (C) Vascularized glioblastoma-on-a-chip was developed and showed the potential for application in personalized medicine [63], copyright (2019) reproduced with permission of Springer Nature.

was associated with superior tumor killing. The results indicate its applicability as mechanistic study and drug-testing platforms.

Remarkably, the ultimate goal of *in vitro* modeling of BVs is to recapitulate the complete functional performance of an organ. The 3D bioprinting technology has demonstrated its potential in vital aspects of vascular tissue engineering to provide ideal models.

6.5 End-of chapter problem and examples

Q1. What are the prerequisites for emulating *in vitro* 3D-engineered tissues/organs?

A. For biomimicry via 3D bioprinting, a practical design should be approached, and the biofabrication strategy should consider the overall architecture of the 3D tissue or *in vitro* 3D platform. The choice of printing material (including cell sources) is essential and specific to the native tissue form and function. Synthetic or natural polymers and tissue-specific dECM are widely used. Furthermore, allogeneic or autologous cell sources have been added to the hydrogel as a bioink and integrated with 3D bioprinting systems. The printed *in vitro* 3D tissues/organs may require a period of maturation in a bioreactor before being utilized for *in vitro* applications such as drug screening and testing.

Q2. Which factors should be considered when evaluating the performance of BVs *in vitro* using 3D bioprinting technology?

A. To elucidate the performance of BVs *in vitro* using 3D bioprinting, multiple factors should be considered, such as biomaterials, including multiple cell types and biocompatible bioinks, and the dimensional design of the vascular architecture, cellular alignment, and molecular gradient.

References

[1] Ashammakhi N, Nasiri R, de Barros N R, Tebon P, Thakor J, Goudie M, Shamloo A, Martin M G and Khademhosseini A 2020 Gut-on-a-chip: current progress and future opportunities *Biomaterials* **255** 120196

[2] Kiela P R and Ghishan F K 2016 Physiology of intestinal absorption and secretion *Best Pract. Res. Cl Ga* **30** 145–59

[3] Han H, Park Y, Choi Y M, Yong U, Kang B, Shin W, Min S, Kim H J, Jang J and Bioprinted A 2022 Tubular intestine model using a colon-specific extracellular matrix bioink *Adv. Healthc. Mater.* **11** e2101768

[4] Stecher B 2015 The roles of inflammation, nutrient availability and the commensal microbiota in enteric pathogen infection *Microbiol. Spectr.* **3** 3.3.12

[5] Lin L and Zhang J Q 2017 Role of intestinal microbiota and metabolites on gut homeostasis and human diseases *BMC Immunol.* **18** 2

[6] Cheng L, Liu T, Lian L, Tang G, Mille L S, García F R, Engstrand L, Zhang Y S and Du J 2023 3D-bioprinted gut anaerobic model for studying bacteria-host interactions *Research* **6** 0058

[7] Du B, Yu M and Zheng J 2018 Transport and interactions of nanoparticles in the kidneys *Nat. Rev. Mater.* **3** 358–74

[8] Smith H W and Beyenbach K W 1996 *The Kidney: Structure and Function in Health and Disease* (Blackwell Science)

[9] Jarad G and Miner J H 2009 Update on the glomerular filtration barrier *Curr. Opin. Nephrol. Hypertens.* **18** 226–32

[10] Eremina V, Baelde H J and Quaggin S E 2007 Role of the VEGF-A signaling pathway in the glomerulus: evidence for crosstalk between components of the glomerular filtration barrier *Nephron. Physiol.* **106** 32–7

[11] Haraldsson B, Nystrom J and Deen W M 2008 Properties of the glomerular barrier and mechanisms of proteinuria *Physiol. Rev.* **88** 451–87

[12] Reitsma S, Slaaf D W, Vink H, van Zandvoort M A M J and Egbrink M G A O 2007 The endothelial glycocalyx: composition, functions, and visualization *Pflug. Arch. Eur. J. Phy.* **454** 345–59

[13] Bishop J H, Green R and Thomas S 1978 Effects of glucose on water and sodium reabsorption in the proximal convoluted tubule of rat kidney *J. Physiol.* **275** 481–93

[14] Imai M and Kokko J P 1976 Mechanism of sodium and chloride transport in the thin ascending limb of Henle *J. Clin. Invest.* **58** 1054–60

[15] Knepper M and Burg M 1983 Organization of nephron function *Am. J. Physiol.* **244** F579–89

[16] Homan K A, Kolesky D B, Skylar-Scott M A, Herrmann J, Obuobi H, Moisan A and Lewis J A 2016 Bioprinting of 3D convoluted renal proximal tubules on perfusable chips *Sci. Rep.* **6** 34845

[17] Ligresti G *et al* 2016 Three-dimensional human peritubular microvascular system *J. Am. Soc. Nephrol.* **27** 2370–81

[18] Lin N Y C, Homan K A, Robinson S S, Kolesky D B, Duarte N, Moisan A and Lewis J A 2019 Renal reabsorption in 3D vascularized proximal tubule models *Proc. Natl Acad. Sci. USA* **116** 5399–404

[19] Singh N K, Han W, Nam S A, Kim J W, Kim J Y, Kim Y K and Cho D W 2020 Three-dimensional cell-printing of advanced renal tubular tissue analogue *Biomaterials* **232** 119734

[20] Singh N K, Kim J Y, Lee J Y, Lee H, Gao G, Jang J, Kim Y K and Cho D W 2023 Coaxial cell printing of a human glomerular model: an *in vitro* glomerular filtration barrier and its pathophysiology *Biofabrication* **15** 024101

[21] Selistre L D S, Cochat P, Rech D L, Parant F, Souza V C and Dubourg L 2018 Association between glomerular filtration rate (measured by high-performance liquid chromatography with iohexol) and plasma oxalate *J. Bras. Nefrol.* **40** 73–6

[22] Bhasin B, Ürekli H M and Atta M G 2015 Primary and secondary hyperoxaluria: understanding the enigma *World J. Nephrol.* **4** 235–44

[23] Mitchell T, Kumar P, Reddy T, Wood K D, Knight J, Assimos D G and Holmes R P 2019 Dietary oxalate and kidney stone formation *Am. J. Physiol. Renal Physiol.* **316** F409–13

[24] Yoon J, Singh N K, Jang J and Cho D-W 2022 3D bioprinted *in vitro* secondary hyperoxaluria model by mimicking intestinal-oxalate-malabsorption-related kidney stone disease *Appl. Phys. Rev.* **9** 041408

[25] Kanitakis J 2002 Anatomy, histology and immunohistochemistry of normal human skin *Eur. J. Dermatol.* **12** 390–400

[26] Kolarsick P, Kolarsick M A and Goodwin C 2011 Anatomy and physiology of the skin *J. Dermatol. Nurses' Assoc.* **3** 203–13

[27] Hudson T J 2006 Skin barrier function and allergic risk *Nat. Genet.* **38** 399–400

[28] Driskell R R and Watt F M 2015 Understanding fibroblast heterogeneity in the skin *Trends Cell Biol.* **25** 92–9

[29] Hansen K and Khanna C 2004 Spontaneous and genetically engineered animal models; use in preclinical cancer drug development *Eur. J. Cancer* **40** 858–80

[30] Liebsch M, Grune B, Seiler A, Butzke D, Oelgeschlager M, Pirow R, Adler S, Riebeling C and Luch A 2011 Alternatives to animal testing: current status and future perspectives *Arch. Toxicol.* **85** 841–58

[31] Doke S K and Dhawale S C 2015 Alternatives to animal testing: a review *Saudi Pharm. J.* **23** 223–9

[32] Xue M and Jackson C J 2015 Extracellular matrix reorganization during wound healing and its impact on abnormal scarring *Adv. Wound Care* **4** 119–36

[33] Kim B S, Gao G, Kim J Y and Cho D W 2019 3D cell printing of perfusable vascularized human skin equivalent composed of epidermis, dermis, and hypodermis for better structural recapitulation of native skin *Adv. Healthc. Mater.* **8** e1801019

[34] Pellegrini G, Dellambra E, Golisano O, Martinelli E, Fantozzi I, Bondanza S, Ponzin D, McKeon F and De M 2001 Luca, p63 identifies keratinocyte stem cells *Proc. Natl. Acad. Sci.* **98** 3156–61

[35] Michel M, Török N, Godbout M J, Lussier M, Gaudreau P, Royal A and Germain L 1996 Keratin 19 as a biochemical marker of skin stem cells *in vivo* and *in vitro*: keratin 19 expressing cells are differentially localized in function of anatomic sites, and their number varies with donor age and culture stage *J. Cell Sci.* **109** 1017–28

[36] Kim B S, Ahn M, Cho W W, Gao G, Jang J and Cho D W 2021 Engineering of diseased human skin equivalent using 3D cell printing for representing pathophysiological hallmarks of type 2 diabetes *in vitro Biomaterials* **272** 120776

[37] Perez M I and Kohn S R 1994 Cutaneous manifestations of diabetes-mellitus *J. Am. Acad. Dermatol.* **30** 519–31

[38] Stumvoll M, Goldstein B J and van Haeften T W 2005 Type 2 diabetes: principles of pathogenesis and therapy *Lancet* **365** 1333–46

[39] Brem H and Tomic-Canic M 2007 Cellular and molecular basis of wound healing in diabetes *J. Clin. Invest.* **117** 1219–22

[40] Kolesky D B, Homan K A, Skylar-Scott M A and Lewis J A 2016 Three-dimensional bioprinting of thick vascularized tissues *Proc. Natl. Acad. Sci.* **113** 3179–84

[41] Luo L and Liu M 2016 Adipose tissue in control of metabolism *J. Endocrinol.* **231** R77–99

[42] Mohamed-Ali V, Pinkney J H and Coppack S W 1998 Adipose tissue as an endocrine and paracrine organ *Int. J. Obes. Relat. Metab. Disord.* **22** 1145–58

[43] Coelho M, Oliveira T and Fernandes R 2013 Biochemistry of adipose tissue: an endocrine organ *Arch. Med. Sci.* **9** 191–200

[44] Sun S, Ji Y, Kersten S and Qi L 2012 Mechanisms of inflammatory responses in obese adipose tissue *Annu. Rev. Nutr.* **32** 261–86

[45] Frühbeck G 2008 Overview of adipose tissue and its role in obesity and metabolic disorders *Methods Mol. Biol.* **456** 1–22

[46] Wisse B E 2004 The inflammatory syndrome: the role of adipose tissue cytokines in metabolic disorders linked to obesity *J. Am. Soc. Nephrol.* **15** 2792–800

[47] Ahn M, Cho W W, Kim B S and Cho D W 2022 Engineering densely packed adipose tissue via environmentally controlled in-bath 3D bioprinting *Adv. Funct. Mater.* **32**

[48] Zhu J, He J, Verano M, Brimmo A T, Glia A, Qasaimeh M A, Chen P, Aleman J O and Chen W 2018 An integrated adipose-tissue-on-chip nanoplasmonic biosensing platform for investigating obesity-associated inflammation *Lab Chip* **18** 3550–60

[49] Pedersen D J *et al* 2015 A major role of insulin in promoting obesity-associated adipose tissue inflammation *Mol. Metab.* **4** 507–18

[50] Humphrey J D and Schwartz M A 2021 Vascular mechanobiology: homeostasis, adaptation, and disease *Annu. Rev. Biomed. Eng.* **23** 1–27

[51] Devillard C D and Marquette C A 2021 Vascular tissue engineering: challenges and requirements for an ideal large scale blood vessel *Front. Bioeng. Biotechnol.* **9** 721843

[52] Lust S T, Shanahan C M, Shipley R J, Lamata P and Gentleman E 2021 Design considerations for engineering 3D models to study vascular pathologies *in vitro Acta Biomater.* **132** 114–28

[53] Cho W-W, Park W, Cho D-W and Yi H-G 2023 Tumour-on-a-chip *Principles of Human Organs-on-Chips* (Elsevier) pp 429–59

[54] Kong Z and Wang X 2023 Bioprinting technologies and bioinks for vascular model establishment *Int. J. Mol. Sci.* **24** 891

[55] Wu W, DeConinck A and Lewis J A 2011 Omnidirectional printing of 3D microvascular networks *Adv. Mater.* **23** H178–83

[56] Gauvin-Rossignol G, Legros P, Ruel J, Fortin M-A and Bégin-Drolet A 2018 Sugar glass fugitive ink loaded with calcium chloride for the rapid casting of alginate scaffold designs *Heliyon* **4** e00680

[57] Song K H, Highley C B, Rouff A and Burdick J A 2018 Complex 3D-printed microchannels within cell-degradable hydrogels *Adv. Funct. Mater.* **28** 1801331

[58] Grigoryan B, Paulsen S J, Corbett D C, Sazer D W, Fortin C L, Zaita A J, Greenfield P T, Calafat N J, Gounley J P and Ta A H 2019 Multivascular networks and functional intravascular topologies within biocompatible hydrogels *Science* **364** 458–64

[59] Gao G, Park J Y, Kim B S, Jang J and Cho D W 2018 Coaxial cell printing of freestanding, perfusable, and functional *in vitro* vascular models for recapitulation of native vascular endothelium pathophysiology *Adv. Healthcare Mater.* **7** 1801102

[60] Gao G, Park W, Kim B S, Ahn M, Chae S, Cho W W, Kim J, Lee J Y, Jang J and Cho D W 2021 Construction of a novel *in vitro* atherosclerotic model from geometry-tunable artery equivalents engineered via in-bath coaxial cell printing *Adv. Funct. Mater.* **31** 2008878

[61] Kim B S, Cho W W, Gao G, Ahn M, Kim J and Cho D W 2021 Construction of tissue-level cancer-vascular model with high-precision position control via *in situ* 3D cell printing *Small Methods* **5** 2100072

[62] Cho W W, Ahn M, Kim B S and Cho D W 2022 Blood-lymphatic integrated system with heterogeneous melanoma spheroids via in-bath three-dimensional bioprinting for modelling of combinational targeted therapy *Adv. Sci.* **9** 2202093

[63] Yi H-G, Jeong Y H, Kim Y, Choi Y-J, Moon H E, Park S H, Kang K S, Bae M, Jang J and Youn H 2019 A bioprinted human-glioblastoma-on-a-chip for the identification of patient-specific responses to chemoradiotherapy *Nat. Biomed. Eng.* **3** 509–19

[64] Park W, Bae M, Hwang M, Jang J, Cho D-W and Yi H-G 2021 3D cell-printed hypoxic cancer-on-a-chip for recapitulating pathologic progression of solid cancer *J. Vis. Exp.* https://www.jove.com/v/61945/3d-cell-printed-hypoxic-cancer-on-chip-for-recapitulating-pathologic

Chapter 7

Future perspective and conclusion

Organ printing technology has innovatively progressed over the past few decades with the aim of creating functional organs that can be integrated into the human body [1]. In particular, current population aging has increased the demand for effective regenerative medicines, which has accelerated the development of organ printing technology. Since the late 1990s, when the first trial to create and implant laboratory-grown human bladders was conducted, researchers have explored the use of tissue engineering technology, especially 3D bioprinting, to reconstitute a wide range of human organs, including bones, eyes, heart, skin, liver, brain, lungs, airways, kidneys, muscles, and blood vessels [2–7]. Owing to its flexibility and versatility, this technology has bridged the gap between engineered tissue constructs and natural tissues by providing a tool for understanding basic physiology and disease development, drug screening, and developing personalized medicines [8]. Therefore, its potential to save lives has been demonstrated through both preclinical and clinical applications.

By focusing on emulating the cellular, biochemical, and mechanical performances of native tissues, artificial tissue equivalents have been developed through a variety of pioneering approaches for regenerative medicine and pharmaceutical research. Moreover, the strategies are based on analyses of process parameters, including the design of nozzles and cartridges, selection of bioprocessable bioinks, sophistication of fabrication strategies, utilization of multi-bioink and multiscale hybrid bioprinting processes, and enhancement of tissue maturation strategy [9]. Although many creative strategies have been suggested to enhance functionalities, including precise controllability and repeatability, for the construction of complex structures, the technology is still in its infancy, and further technological improvements are needed.

More insights into the systemic investigation of organ printing technology are required for successful future research. Dynamic coupling of biological, chemical, physical, and computational approaches should be performed to build 3D functional tissue constructs [10]. Based on a better understanding of complex cellular signaling pathways, the study of cross-organ communications, including regulatory

doi:10.1088/978-0-7503-5122-5ch7

pathways or hormonal feedback loops, as well as the study of single organs, will be possible [11]. Moreover, the development of stimuli-responsive-material-combined four-dimensional printing technology will enable the programmable self-assembly of tissue and organ constructions and allow the investigation of the developmental and morphological change-associated functions of human organs [12]. Furthermore, high-resolution and high-speed imaging technologies must be developed. More importantly, integration and standardization at each step are required for successful technological innovation. If this is achieved, organ printing will become the next-generation core technology for the production of complex human tissues/organs for clinical translation.

References

[1] He J, Mao M, Li X and Chua C K 2021 Bioprinting of 3D functional tissue constructs *Int. J. Bioprint.* **7** 395

[2] Bae M, Ko M K, Jin Y, Shin W J, Park W, Chae S, Lee H J, Jang J, Yi H-G and Lee D S 2021 Neural stem cell delivery using brain-derived tissue-specific bioink for recovering from traumatic brain injury *Biofabrication* **13** 044110

[3] Park W, Gao G and Cho D-W 2021 Tissue-specific decellularized extracellular matrix bioinks for musculoskeletal tissue regeneration and modeling using 3D bioprinting technology *Int. J. Mol. Sci.* **22** 7837

[4] Gao G, Park W, Kim B S, Ahn M, Chae S, Cho W W, Kim J, Lee J Y, Jang J and Cho D W 2021 Construction of a novel *in vitro* atherosclerotic model from geometry-tunable artery equivalents engineered via in-bath coaxial cell printing *Adv. Funct. Mater.* **31** 2008878

[5] Park J H, Ahn M, Park S H, Kim H, Bae M, Park W, Hollister S J, Kim S W and Cho D-W 2021 3D bioprinting of a trachea-mimetic cellular construct of a clinically relevant size *Biomaterials* **279** 121246

[6] Park W, Bae M, Hwang M, Jang J, Cho D-W and Yi H-G 2021 3D cell-printed hypoxic cancer-on-a-chip for recapitulating pathologic progression of solid cancer *J. Vis. Exp.* https://www.jove.com/v/61945/3d-cell-printed-hypoxic-cancer-on-chip-for-recapitulating-pathologic

[7] Chae S, Yong U, Park W, Choi Y-m, Jeon I-H, Kang H, Jang J, Choi H S and Cho D-W 2023 3D cell-printing of gradient multi-tissue interfaces for rotator cuff regeneration *Bioact. Mater.* **19** 611–25

[8] Yi H-G, Kim H, Kwon J, Choi Y-J, Jang J and Cho D-W 2021 Application of 3D bioprinting in the prevention and the therapy for human diseases *Signal Transduct. Target. Therapy* **6** 177

[9] Cho D-W, Lee J-S, Jang J, Jung J W, Park J H and Pati F 2015 *Organ Printing* (Morgan & Claypool Publishers)

[10] Dinh J-L, Godin C and Azpeitia E 2022 Introduction to computational modeling of multicellular tissues *Plant Systems Biology: Methods and Protocols* (Berlin: Springer) pp 107–45

[11] Picollet-D'hahan N, Zuchowska A, Lemeunier I and Le Gac S 2021 Multiorgan-on-a-chip: a systemic approach to model and decipher inter-organ communication *Trends Biotechnol.* **39** 788–810

[12] Ahmed A, Arya S, Gupta V, Furukawa H and Khosla A 2021 4D printing: fundamentals, materials, applications and challenges *Polymer* **228** 123926

www.ingramcontent.com/pod-product-compliance
Ingram Content Group UK Ltd.
Pitfield, Milton Keynes, MK11 3LW, UK
UKHW051848100926
8556IPUK00005B/510

9 780750 351201